KT-103-216

# Coping with Endometriosis

Jill Eckersley is a freelance writer with many years' experience of writing on health topics. She is a regular contributor to women's and general-interest magazines, including *Women's Running*, *Women's Fitness* and other titles. She is the author of many other books for Sheldon Press, including *Coping with Childhood Asthma*, *Helping Children Cope with Anxiety*, *Every Woman's Guide to Heart Health*, *Every Woman's Guide to Digestive Health*, *Coping with Early-onset Dementia* and *Helping Elderly Relatives*, all published between 2003 and 2013. She lives beside the Regent's Canal in north London with her cat.

Dr Zara Aziz is a GP working in a large and busy urban practice in Bristol. She has interests in cardiovascular health, family medicine and disease prevention. She is involved in medical education and trains junior doctors to become GPs. She is a keen medical writer and writes for a number of publications, including a 'Doctor's orders' column for *The Guardian*. She is the author, with Dr Shahid Aziz, of *Understanding High Blood Pressure* (Sheldon Press, 2014).

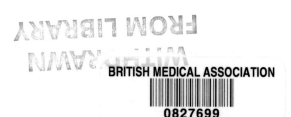

FROM LIBRARY
WITHDRAWN

BRITISH MEDICAL ASSOCIATION
0827699

# Overcoming Common Problems Series

*Selected titles*

A full list of titles is available from Sheldon Press,
36 Causton Street, London SW1P 4ST and on our website at
www.sheldonpress.co.uk

**Breast Cancer: Your treatment choices**
Dr Terry Priestman

**Chronic Fatigue Syndrome: What you need
to know about CFS/ME**
Dr Megan A. Arroll

**Cider Vinegar**
Margaret Hills

**Coeliac Disease: What you need to know**
Alex Gazzola

**Coping Successfully with Hiatus Hernia**
Dr Tom Smith

**Coping with Difficult Families**
Dr Jane McGregor and Tim McGregor

**Coping with Epilepsy**
Dr Pamela Crawford and Fiona Marshall

**Coping with Memory Problems**
Dr Sallie Baxendale

**Coping with the Psychological Effects
of Illness**
Dr Fran Smith, Dr Carina Eriksen
and Professor Robert Bor

**Coping with Schizophrenia**
Professor Kevin Gournay and Debbie Robson

**Coping with Thyroid Disease**
Mark Greener

**Depressive Illness: The curse of the strong**
Dr Tim Cantopher

**Dr Dawn's Guide to Brain Health**
Dr Dawn Harper

**Dr Dawn's Guide to Heart Health**
Dr Dawn Harper

**Dr Dawn's Guide to Weight and Diabetes**
Dr Dawn Harper

**Dr Dawn's Guide to Women's Health**
Dr Dawn Harper

**The Empathy Trap: Understanding
antisocial personalities**
Dr Jane McGregor and Tim McGregor

**The Fibromyalgia Healing Diet**
Christine Craggs-Hinton

**Fibromyalgia: Your treatment guide**
Christine Craggs-Hinton

**Helping Elderly Relatives**
Jill Eckersley

**The Holistic Health Handbook**
Mark Greener

**How to Stop Worrying**
Dr Frank Tallis

**Invisible Illness: Coping with
misunderstood conditions**
Dr Megan A. Arroll and Professor
Christine P. Dancey

**Living with the Challenges of Dementia:
A guide for family and friends**
Patrick McCurry

**Living with Complicated Grief**
Professor Craig A. White

**Living with Fibromyalgia**
Christine Craggs-Hinton

**Living with Hearing Loss**
Dr Don McFerran, Lucy Handscomb
and Dr Cherilee Rutherford

**Overcoming Fear with Mindfulness**
Deborah Ward

**Overcoming Low Self-esteem with Mindfulness**
Deborah Ward

**Overcoming Stress**
Professor Robert Bor, Dr Carina Eriksen
and Dr Sara Chaudry

**Overcoming Worry and Anxiety**
Dr Jerry Kennard

**Physical Intelligence: How to take charge
of your weight**
Dr Tom Smith

**Post-Traumatic Stress Disorder: Recovery after
accident and disaster**
Professor Kevin Gournay

**The Self-Esteem Journal**
Alison Waines

**The Stroke Survival Guide**
Mark Greener

**Ten Steps to Positive Living**
Dr Windy Dryden

**Treating Arthritis: The drug-free way**
Margaret Hills and Christine Horner

**Understanding High Blood Pressure**
Dr Shahid Aziz and Dr Zara Aziz

**Understanding Yourself and Others: Practical
ideas from the world of coaching**
Bob Thomson

**When Someone You Love Has Depression:
A handbook for family and friends**
Barbara Baker

Overcoming Common Problems

# Coping with Endometriosis

JILL ECKERSLEY
and
DR ZARA AZIZ

**sheldon** PRESS

First published in Great Britain in 2015

Sheldon Press
36 Causton Street
London SW1P 4ST
www.sheldonpress.co.uk

Copyright © Jill Eckersley and Dr Zara Aziz 2015
Foreword copyright © Hilary Mantel 2015

All rights reserved. No part of this book may be reproduced or
transmitted in any form or by any means, electronic or mechanical,
including photocopying, recording, or by any information storage and
retrieval system, without permission in writing from the publisher.

The author and publisher have made every effort to ensure that the
external website and email addresses included in this book are correct and
up to date at the time of going to press. The author and publisher are not
responsible for the content, quality or continuing accessibility of the sites.

*British Library Cataloguing-in-Publication Data*
A catalogue record for this book is available from the British Library

ISBN 978–1–84709–352–3
eBook ISBN 978–1–84709–353–0

Typeset by Fakenham Prepress Solutions, Fakenham, Norfolk NR21 8NN
First printed in Great Britain by Ashford Colour Press
Subsequently digitally reprinted in Great Britain

eBook by Fakenham Prepress Solutions, Fakenham, Norfolk NR21 8NN

Produced on paper from sustainable forests

# Contents

# Foreword

When a woman is first given a diagnosis of endometriosis, or when she first suspects that this puzzling condition may be the reason for her ill-health, what she needs is a friend: a well-informed, plain-speaking guide, who can suggest what she should do next and assure her that she is not alone. This book, I believe, is that friend and guide. Practical and easy to understand, it will help not only women with endometriosis but also their partners and family. I hope, too, that it will reach GPs and nurses, as it pulls together so many useful facts in a concise way. There are many myths about this condition, and professionals are not immune to the effect of them.

For many years, endometriosis sufferers were ignored and stig-matized. It was labelled 'the career women's disease', afflicting those who supposedly were too selfish to have their babies young. Imagine the anger and distress this stigma caused, among women who would have loved to have children . . . if the condition itself didn't hinder them. The myth was that endometriosis did not affect women till they were in their thirties, which was tough if, like me, you had your first symptoms with your first period.

My own battle with the disorder seems to have occupied most of my life. Period pains were normal, I was told, and if I seemed to suffer more than most, it must be because I had a 'low pain threshold'. At 19, I began actively seeking a diagnosis. I was 27 when I received it, and by that time, major surgery was the only answer. Abruptly I lost my fertility and, in some ways, lost myself; though I was told I was cured, the condition recurred, and drug treatment led to huge weight gain: thyroid failure followed, and the devastating chain of consequences pursues me to this day. Anything I have achieved has been in the teeth of the disease.

It need not be like this. My story is extreme and points to the need for early diagnosis. Women of any age need the courage to come forward and ask for help, and health practitioners, teachers and parents need to listen. The condition is not easy to diagnose, because its effects are so diverse and so individual, and because the intensity of pain does not necessarily relate to the severity of the condition. Each case needs to be handled individually, and the patient may have to make some difficult choices. Here, too, this book can help, with a survey of the latest treatments. It is important at every stage to ask questions, and to seek second opinions if necessary. If your doctor sees you as a statistic, or a file to be processed, walk away; you are too precious for that. Your strengths and resources, as well as your pains, are yours alone. Curious, compassionate doctors are out there, in increasing numbers. You may need to be persistent, as this book's case histories show; but there are many avenues to healing, and often a happy outcome.

A few of those avenues are explored in the section on self-help and complementary therapy. Exhortations to eat up your greens and go to the gym can seem insulting to women struggling to keep food inside them or get to work on time, and it is hard even for sensitive people, if their own health is sound, to imagine the daily botches and compromises that people in pain make to keep themselves going. But when it is possible, we should treat our body as a healthy body and respect it; and on good days, invest in it, build its resources. If you exercise, the authors say, put some thought into finding an activity you like. And when looking for help, be open-minded. Alternative practitioners are often good listeners and highly empathetic. From my own experience I know that, if you have been stressed by rushed consultations and tick-box methods, simply to speak and be heard is beneficial. Herbal medicine harnesses the knowledge of countless generations gone before us. Reflexology, autogenic training – a range of therapies can help with pain control, with the side effects of drug treatment, and with self-image. Women with endometriosis often lose their confidence, and carry a burden of sadness that longs for release. Kind people and safe spaces are what we all need. There is no one way of experiencing this condition, and no one way of coping with it. Whatever brings comfort is valid. Whatever works is to be valued.

I would like to believe cases like mine could not occur nowadays. But I fear they will, till there is official awareness of the cost of ignoring this condition – the cost to sufferers, their families, the wider economic community. Endometriosis is not easy to talk about. It cannot be explained in a phrase. It doesn't show on the outside. It touches on areas of women's experience we are sometimes ashamed to speak of. But we must find a way to voice our needs, if we are to command resources for research, if we are to understand and overcome endometriosis, and find a way of coping till we are free from it. This book, I think, will help us to speak.

*Dame Hilary Mantel*

*Dame Hilary Mantel is a writer who has twice won the Man Booker prize for fiction, and recently began a new career as a playwright, receiving a joint Tony nomination for her first efforts on Broadway. She began to suffer from endometriosis when she was 11, was diagnosed at 27, has battled the condition since and has survived it to recover good health.*

# Acknowledgements

I could not have written this book without the help of the many clinicians, researchers and therapists who generously shared their time and expertise with me. They include gynaecologists Michael Dooley, Bini Ajay, Alfred Cutner, Christian Becker, Krina Zondervan, Caroline Overton, Andrew Horne and researcher Nicola Tempest, as well as homoeopath Mollie Hunton, acupuncturist Judy Elliott, herbalist Hananja Brice-Ytsma, reflexologist Tracey Smith, natural health expert Maryon Stewart, hypnotherapist Anne Lee and Relate counsellor Denise Knowles. Special thanks are due to Endometriosis UK's trustee Carol Pearson, who set me on the right road! And – perhaps most vital of all – the many women living with endometriosis who shared their stories with me. Thank you all.

*Jill Eckersley*

# Note to the reader

This is not a medical book and is not intended to replace advice from your doctor. Consult your pharmacist or doctor if you believe you have any of the symptoms described, and if you think you might need medical help.

# Introduction

Endometriosis is an extremely common and very painful gynae-cological condition affecting roughly one in ten women of reproductive age, which means it affects around one and a half million women in the UK and an estimated 176 million world-wide. Astonishingly, endometriosis has been under-researched, under-funded and under-diagnosed until recently, even though the symptoms – excruciatingly painful periods, bowel and bladder problems, extreme fatigue – were first described in a medical treatise as long ago as 1690! There does seem to be an increase in the inci-dence of endometriosis these days, perhaps because women in the twenty-first century don't spend as much of their time either preg-nant or breastfeeding as women did in the past. By the 1920s, there had only been about 20 mentions of endometriosis in medical literature. At that time a Dr John Sampson, writing a research paper in 1927, described 13 cases of endometriosis which he had observed during abdominal surgery.

Even today, it is quite common for women to have to wait several years – up to 20 in some cases – to obtain a diagnosis. This is often because many women still think of period pain as 'normal' and 'just part of being a woman', and don't take their worries to their GP. If they do, it can be difficult for a busy GP to distinguish between the symptoms of endometriosis and the symptoms of other condi-tions, such as irritable bowel syndrome (IBS), which can also cause pelvic pain. However, more and more women are beginning to realize that being crippled with pain, either for a few days every month or most of the time, is anything but normal. Through the pioneering work of a handful of researchers and of support groups, such as Endometriosis UK, awareness is increasing and more funds are being put into research into the causes of, and possible treatments for, endometriosis.

# 1

# What is endometriosis?

Ruby – whose story concludes in Chapter 9 – was diagnosed with endometriosis after many years of pain and discomfort, a situation which is, still, all too common.

I always had terribly painful periods, right from the start when I was 12. Mum took me to the doctor but I never felt that the problem was taken seriously, or that I was listened to. After all, most girls get period pains, don't they? One doctor even told me it was just growing pains. I would be doubled over and crying with the pain. Sometimes I could hardly walk. I felt sick, exhausted and had no energy. When I was eventually referred to a gynaecologist I was told I had Stage IV endometriosis – the most serious kind – and that it was all over my pelvic area, bowel and back.

During my twenties I had 15 stays in hospital and 13 operations, but they never seemed to get to the root of the problem. In-between, I was given some of the heavy-duty drugs which are used to treat the condition but they had awful side effects. At one point my weight went up from nine and a half to 15 stone. I had to have a monthly injection which put me through a premature menopause. I started to look like a bodybuilder and hardly recognized myself. I would be drenched in sweat and had such serious mood swings I felt like killing someone. Another drug I was prescribed gave me acne all over my body. Not surprisingly, I lost all my confidence, especially after I had an ectopic pregnancy caused by endometriosis in my Fallopian tubes. By the time I was 30 all the doctors could offer me was a total hysterectomy, until I saw one gynaecologist who suggested I try complementary therapies.

Endometriosis is the second most common gynaecological condition, after fibroids, in the UK. So if you have just been diagnosed, you are certainly not alone. But what exactly is it?

Endometriosis is a condition in which tissue very similar to the endometrium, or womb lining, grows in other parts of the body. It is most commonly found in the pelvic area, but can also be found elsewhere; for example, in the chest or lungs. We shall be looking at the possible causes for this in Chapter 3.

In the correct place – inside the womb – the endometrium reacts to monthly hormonal fluctuations to produce a monthly period, as the womb lining is shed when no pregnancy occurs. Endometriosis behaves in just the same way and produces a bleed, but this blood has nowhere to go. The result can be inflammation, scarring, adhesions (where internal organs are fused together), cysts, and small lumps or nodules, all of which are affected by the natural monthly hormone changes in your body. This can cause excruciating pain and the other symptoms described in Chapter 2.

## Your menstrual cycle

It can help to understand endometriosis if you know exactly how your menstrual cycle really works, and how hormones affect your reproductive organs. Your cycle is controlled by a part of your brain called the hypothalamus, which produces a hormone called gonadotrophin-releasing hormone (GnRH). This stimulates the pituitary gland at the base of the brain which, in its turn, produces follicle-stimulating hormone (FSH) to ripen an egg each month. It also produces luteinizing hormone (LH) which triggers ovulation, or the release of the egg from the ovary. The egg then travels down the Fallopian tube to the womb, which is lined with endometrial tissue, blood and mucus. Hormones produced by the ovaries, such as oestrogen and progesterone, ensure that the endometrium expands to about ten times its normal thickness every month, to provide nutrients for a fertilized egg and nourish a growing baby. Of course, when there is no fertilized egg and no growing baby, the thickened endometrium breaks up and passes out of the body as the monthly period.

For most healthy women, this completely natural process is not too troublesome, although most of us do experience either the mood swings of pre-menstrual syndrome (PMS) or some discomfort – or both – around period time! However, if you have endometriosis, it means that endometrial cells have migrated from your womb to other parts of your body. Like the womb lining, they react to these normal monthly hormone fluctuations, thickening up and becoming engorged with blood. This can irritate surrounding tissue and, depending where in the body it is found, can interfere with the normal functioning of the reproductive organs, bladder and bowel, as well as causing severe cramping pains.

Endometriosis is most commonly found in the pelvic area – affecting the womb and the surrounding ligaments, the ovaries and Fallopian tubes, the lining of the pelvis and the top of the vagina (see Figure 1). Endometriosis can vary widely in size, shape and colour, and can both shrink or grow over the years. In the earliest stages it can look like pimples, then later be seen as flat areas or lesions. Sometimes it forms small nodules, or what are called chocolate cysts, on or in the ovaries, which are filled with old blood, and can range in size between a pea and a grapefruit! Endometriosis may cause dark-coloured spots or scar tissue, or filmy, web-like adhesions which can stick your organs together. Some of these cause pain, others don't – which is one of the reasons endometriosis is difficult to diagnose.

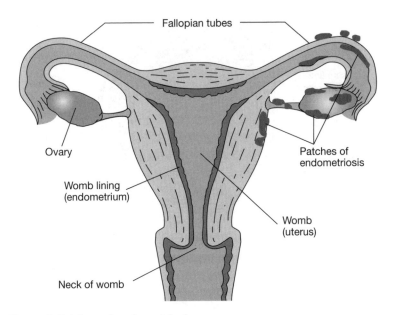

**Figure 1 Patches of endometriosis**

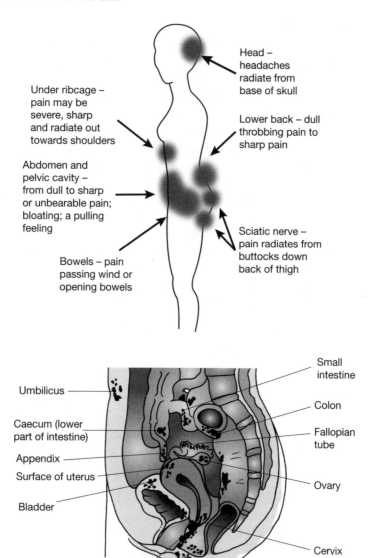

Head – headaches radiate from base of skull

Under ribcage – pain may be severe, sharp and radiate out towards shoulders

Lower back – dull throbbing pain to sharp pain

Abdomen and pelvic cavity – from dull to sharp or unbearable pain; bloating; a pulling feeling

Sciatic nerve – pain radiates from buttocks down back of thigh

Bowels – pain passing wind or opening bowels

Umbilicus

Small intestine

Colon

Caecum (lower part of intestine)

Fallopian tube

Appendix

Surface of uterus

Ovary

Bladder

Cervix

Vagina  Vulva

**Figure 2 Common sites of endometriosis**

*Endometriosis myth – the worse the pain, the worse your condition*

So, contrary to common perception, you can't judge how bad your endometriosis is by how bad your pain is, which is a major source of frustration for many women. That is, there doesn't seem to be a direct link between the severity of the endometriosis, and the amount of pain it produces. So, for example, you might be told you have mild endometriosis, but suffer severe pain – conversely, some women have severe endometriosis but little pain. The pain involved largely depends on where in your body the scars, adhesions or nodules are. (See Chapter 2 for more on pain and other symptoms.)

Areas of the body that can be affected by endometriosis (see Figure 2) include:

- the ovaries and Fallopian tubes
- the outside of the womb
- the area between the rectum (back passage) and womb
- the peritoneum (the thin layer of tissue lining the inside of the abdomen)
- the bowel or bladder
- the vagina and/or rectum
- scars from previous operations
- rarely, the skin, eyes, spine, lungs or brain.

## Fertility

As, in many women, much of the endometriosis occurs around the reproductive organs, it is not surprising that there is a link with fertility. It has been estimated that between a third and a half of women who are apparently infertile actually have endometriosis. We shall be looking in detail at the effect of endometriosis on fertility in Chapter 6. It's important to be aware, though, that having endometriosis doesn't automatically mean that you will not be able to have children. Many women can and do.

## Stages of endometriosis

Endometriosis is sometimes classified into different stages depending on its severity, extent and position in the body. A commonly used score is that produced by the American Society for Reproductive Medicine, who classify endometriosis into one of four stages:

- stage I – minimal
- stage II – mild
- stage III – moderate
- stage IV – severe.

Most women have minimal or mild endometriosis. However, this score is used not so much as to measure the severity of endometriosis, but to assess how it affects fertility. (See Chapter 6).

## How endometriosis may affect you

Endometriosis is a highly individual condition. Your symptoms, and the problems they cause, will depend on exactly where in your body the cysts, inflammation and scarring are. For example, in addition to – or instead of – painful periods and worries about your future fertility, you might have problems with your bladder and bowels. There might be pain when you go to the loo or you may have unexplained diarrhoea and/or constipation, which is why some women are wrongly diagnosed with irritable bowel syndrome rather than endometriosis.

Endometriosis can affect women mentally and emotionally, as well as physically. Dealing with chronic pain can be wearing. Partners, friends, family, employers and workmates are not always sympathetic and if you seem to be trailing backwards and forwards to your GP with a variety of unexplained symptoms you can be made to feel like a malingerer. Even other women may not appreciate what you have to go through each month. Endometriosis is more than just a bad period pain.

Endometriosis can also affect your sex life. Depending on where the cysts or adhesions are, they can make sex extremely uncomfortable, even excruciating at some time during your monthly cycle. If you don't have a sympathetic partner, this can make you feel guilty, resentful, or miserable at missing out on what should be a joyful part of your relationship. The only way to deal with this is to talk things though with your partner so that he is, at least, aware of what the problem is. You haven't gone off him, or gone off sex, you have a painful medical condition. There are plenty of other ways to show affection if you don't feel like having intercourse – maybe a gentle massage might soothe the pain? If you're planning a family, concern about whether you will be able to have children can also impact on your relationship. The more you – and your partner – know about endometriosis, the better you will both be able to cope.

### Endometriosis myths

It's important, too, to be aware of what endometriosis is *not*.

- Although endometriosis can make you feel miserable, it is not fatal.
- It is not infectious or contagious, so no-one else can 'catch' it from you, and you did not catch it from anyone else.
- It is not and is not related to any form of cancer, and endometrial cells in other parts of the body have the same chance of becoming cancerous as any of the body's other cells.
- It is not a 'career woman's problem' – a kind of punishment for working women who have chosen to delay having children until they are in their 30s or later. Most women with endometriosis are between 20 and 45, but it is also found in teenagers and sometimes even in post-menopausal women. According to the SHE Trust (see Useful addresses), the youngest well-documented case was in a 10-year-old who had had just two periods, and the oldest in a post-menopausal woman of 78.
- It is not restricted to women from any particular ethnic background, although some studies have suggested that it is slightly more common in Asian women than white Caucasians, and slightly less common in women from an African Caribbean background.

# 2

# Symptoms

Endometriosis is a chronic or long-term condition, and can be debilitating, affecting your physical and mental well-being. It is not, however, life-threatening, and symptoms can be treated. While a total cure remains elusive, much can be done to lessen pain and improve quality of life.

A great deal depends on where in the body the rogue endometrial cells are and, as we have already seen, the amount of endometriosis you have doesn't always tally with the amount of pain, or other symptoms. You may always have had more painful than average periods, or you may develop symptoms over time. In either case, you should be aware of:

- very heavy or prolonged periods (menorrhagia);

It's worth knowing that the average blood loss during a period is just 30–40 ml. Anything over 60 ml counts as heavy. If your period lasts longer than 7 days, if you often have to use double protection (towel and tampon, or two tampons), if you flood and stain your clothes or bedding or pass large blood clots or feel nervous about going out or wearing light clothes during your period, that counts as heavy or prolonged.

- severe pain in your pelvic area, abdomen, back or legs which is associated with your period, and doesn't respond to ordinary painkillers or 'home remedies', such as hot-water bottles or warm baths. Women with endometriosis commonly talk about being crippled, bent double or unable to stand up straight because of the pain;
- irregular bleeding outside period times, including spotting;
- pelvic pain at other times of the month;
- feeling nauseous or faint at period times, or actually vomiting;
- feeling excessively tired and lacking in energy to the point when

you have to stay in bed and don't feel able to carry on with your normal routine;

- pain during, or after, sex;
- frequent vaginal infections such as thrush;
- difficulty in becoming pregnant even when you are having regular unprotected sex. (For more about endometriosis and fertility, see Chapter 6);
- pain when you use the loo, especially around period time. Any blood in your urine/faeces should always be mentioned to your doctor. Some women get constipation, diarrhoea, right-sided abdominal pain, bladder irritation or urgency or frequent urinary tract infections. Many of these symptoms can be associated with other conditions, such as irritable bowel syndrome, which partly explains why diagnosis can take so long.

Any of these symptoms may be associated with endometriosis and having several symptoms will make a diagnosis more likely. It is a good idea to keep a pain diary so that you can give the medical professionals treating you a full picture of what's happening. A symptom diary can be added to give a clearer picture. For example, it might be easier to work out where the endometriosis is if you can tell the doctor that standing, sitting or lying in a particular position makes the pain feel better, or worse.

### Quick checklist of key symptoms

- Painful and/or heavy periods
- Pain in the lower abdomen, pelvis or lower back
- Pain during and after sex – typically a deep stabbing pain
- Bleeding between periods
- Difficulty getting pregnant
- Ongoing tiredness and exhaustion
- Discomfort when passing water or stools
- Bleeding from the back passage or blood in your stools.

Related problems may include:
- Bloating, abnormal bowel movements and vomiting
- Bowel or urinary disorders associated with periods
- Allergies or migraines that become worse around menstruation.

If you have always had problem periods, it might be difficult for you to know just exactly what is normal and which symptoms suggest that a visit to your GP might be in order. Many teenagers and older women get period cramps, but it's not normal to be crippled by cramps for more than a few hours, or to be prevented from leading a normal life during your periods.

## Distinguishing endometriosis from normal period pain

Period pain is, of course, very common, which is one reason why a diagnosis of endometriosis can take a long time. Just what is normal, and how much discomfort should women be expected to put up with before they seek medical help?

Pain and other period-related symptoms do vary from woman to woman. Some women have cramps caused by the muscular contraction of the walls of the womb. These can compress the blood vessels which line the womb and cut off the blood and/or oxygen supply, causing spasms of pain. Many women describe the pain radiating out across the area between their hips and the tops of their legs (rather than just being confined to the womb). Other women just get a dull, constant ache, sometimes spreading to the back or thighs, which often starts when the bleeding begins and goes on for perhaps 12-24 hours. Some women have pain all the time, while others only have pain during their periods, when they have sex or when they go to the toilet.

To deal with monthly discomfort from period pain, most women find relief from a couple of painkillers, either paracetamol or ibuprofen, or products like Feminax which are specially formulated for period pain. A warm bath, some relaxation exercises, a massage or snuggling up with a hot-water bottle are also traditional ways of coping with the pain.

However, if you find your symptoms are much worse than that, if the pain is really crippling and actually prevents you from carrying on with your normal life for more than a few hours, that could be the time to ask for help. Table 1 is a quick guide to what's to be expected in period pain, and what may indicate endometriosis.

**Table 1 Normal period pain versus endometriosis pain**

| Normal period pain | Endometriosis pain |
| --- | --- |
| is typically felt in the first day or two of a period as cramping | may be felt later on in the period, or before it |
| is usually felt in the lower abdomen where the uterus is | pain may extend right across the abdomen or pelvis, and/or to the lower back or legs |
| may be severe for a few hours or a day but not unbearable | may be very severe, so that it has you doubled up or lying flat |
| usually responds to over-the-counter treatment | cannot be eased by over-the-counter remedies |

## A pain diary

Before you go to the doctor, it can be helpful to keep a pain diary for a few months so that you can give your GP detailed information about what exactly the problems are and when they occur. For example:

- Do you have pain before or during your period or halfway through your cycle? Some unfortunate women have pain virtually all the time and if this is the case for you, then tell your GP.
- Where is the pain – in your pelvic area, back, the back of your legs, your stomach?
- Do you feel nauseous or actually vomit?

Tell the doctor as much about the pain as you can.

- What kind of pain is it, or does it vary?
- Is it a dragging, constant pain, an irregular, cramping pain or more of a dull ache?
- How long does it commonly last?
- Do you feel faint?
- Are you able to carry on with your normal routine or do you have to miss school, college or work for those few days every month?
- Have you tried over-the-counter (OTC) painkillers and have they had any effect?
- How many painkillers do you have to take every day to keep the pain under control, or are you not able to do this?

- Is there anything at all that you have done which does seem to help the pain, such as a heat pack or a warm bath?

Also tell your doctor if you have gastrointestinal symptoms:

- Is there a link to your bladder or bowels? In other words, is going to the loo painful at any time of the month, or all the time?
- Are the symptoms worse if you are constipated?
- Do you get diarrhoea, or alternating constipation and diarrhoea?
- Do you have intestinal cramping or abdominal pain (though this can be hard to differentiate from period pain)?
- Do you have rectal pain or rectal bleeding?

Information like this will help to convince your GP that this is more than just a case of period pain. The more information you can give to health professionals, the easier they will find it to treat you, which may include referring you to a gynaecologist for further investigations. You can even say that you wonder if you might have endometriosis.

The most common symptoms which bring women to the care of a gynaecologist are pelvic pain, pain during intercourse, painful periods and subfertility, according to Bini Ajay, consultant gynae-cologist at Spire St Anthony's Hospital at Cheam in Surrey, who has a special interest in pelvic pain and endometriosis. Observations by Ms Ajay suggest that the diagnosis rate is increasing as women become more aware of the condition, which leads them to see a GP or gynaecologist earlier. In addition, the fact that endometriosis can run in families means that mothers tend to bring their daughters in for medical care earlier.

## *Migraine*

There are several studies to show that women with endometriosis frequently experience migraine – one study showed that around a third of women with endometriosis also had migraine – roughly double the normal level of migraine in the population (around 15 per cent). 'Do seek help for your migraine,' says author Dame Hilary Mantel. 'Because it is outside the gynaecological/gastrointestinal nexus within which women are treated, it is easy for a woman to regard it as just one more thing she has to put up with, or as part of PMS. Whereas in fact it is highly amenable to treatment, and there is nothing to stop a woman asking to be referred to a specialist for it, if she's not getting help from her GP or from over-the-counter medications.

'I think we become apologetic about taking up resources, and asking extra questions. With endometriosis you are not going to get a quick fix, so you have to look for every way possible to make your life better while you are seeking a cure, and that may mean focusing on the bits and pieces you can remedy. The fact is that women with this condition can suffer despair. You need to ask yourself, "What can I do, today/tomorrow/at this very moment, to help myself feel better?" and in that way you can tackle your problems bit by bit, whereas the whole can seem overwhelming.'

# 3

# Causes

The cause of endometriosis is not yet known, although research is ongoing. There are believed to be multiple contributory factors, some of which may be inherited, so it might be worthwhile finding out whether your mother, aunts, older sisters or other family members have had the same problems. One major study from the USA, quoted below, showed that two-thirds of the women with endometriosis studied had relatives also diagnosed with or suspected of having endometriosis. Remember, it may well not have been actually diagnosed in older family members, who may be shy about discussing period problems. Among the current suggestions for the most likely causes are:

- *Retrograde blood flow* This means that instead of leaving the body in the form of a period, some menstrual blood flows backwards down the Fallopian tubes and into the pelvic area. There, endometrial cells from the womb begin to grow on the surface of different pelvic organs and endometriosis develops. However, if this is indeed the case, we don't know why this process only happens in some women and not others, and if so, what makes it happen. It turns out that most women have retrograde blood flow sometimes, but the stray blood does not remain on their organs and is absorbed by the body. So why does that happen? We just don't know. Linked to this is the idea that these rogue endometrial cells might be carried to other parts of the body in blood vessels or via lymph drainage. This would explain why a minority of women have symptoms of endometriosis in other parts of their bodies and not only in the pelvic area. Once again, though, if this happens we don't know why it affects only some women, or how it might actually happen.
- *Metaplasia* This is a process by which perfectly normal cells elsewhere in the body, for example in the ovaries or the lining of the

abdomen, might change into endometrial cells. It is not known why this might happen either.

• *Dysfunction in the immune system* It has been suggested that some women's immune systems are unable to fight the rogue cells, and that endometriosis should be classed as an autoimmune disease in which the body fails to recognize and destroy cells that are growing in the wrong place. One research study found that endometrial tissue found outside the womb contained more T regulatory cells, which can suppress the immune system, than expected so that the body was unable to destroy this tissue. Another suggestion is that the immune system might over-react to the presence of endome-trial cells and produce interleukins (body chemicals which boost the immune system) and prostaglandins (naturally occurring molecules which control processes such as inflammation). These, in their turn, are known to damage tissues. One major study of women in the USA with surgically diagnosed endometriosis, published in 2002 in the journal *Human Reproduction*, suggested that women with endometriosis have a higher than average risk of autoimmune disorders.[1] In some cases, the figures were quite startling. Researchers at the National Institute of Child Health and Human Development, at George Washington University, USA, said that women with endometriosis were:

– twice as likely to have fibromyalgia, characterized by pain in the muscles, joints and tendons;
– 7 times more likely to have hypothyroid problems (under-active thyroid gland);
– 100 times more likely to have Chronic Fatigue Syndrome, with fatigue unrelieved by rest lasting six months or more.

Also, more of those with endometriosis had autoimmune dis-eases such as multiple sclerosis, rheumatoid arthritis, lupus (a condition where the immune system attacks healthy tissue, causing joint and muscle pain and extreme tiredness), Sjögren's syndrome (a condition in which the immune system attacks the tear and salivary glands, causing eye and mouth dryness), asthma and allergies. This does suggest that the immune system might play a role – but are these other conditions actually a cause of endometriosis, or could they be the result of it? At present the jury seems still to be out on that idea.

- *Environmental factors* Exposure to dioxins seems to affect endometriosis in animals, but to date there has been no positive proof that such chemicals are a factor in humans. One recent US study found that there might be a link between endometriosis and exposure to organochlorine pesticides. The researchers had compared several hundred women who had been exposed to these with another similar-sized group who had not, and found that those exposed to the pesticides had a 30–70 per cent higher risk of developing endometriosis. These compounds are now either banned from use in the UK and the EU, or are being phased out.
- *Hormonal factors* Some studies have suggested that women who are exposed to more of the hormone oestrogen – for example, women who start their periods earlier than average and have shorter cycles and longer, heavier periods – might be more likely to have endometriosis. Even if this does prove to be a risk factor, however, many women who start their periods later and have average cycles also have endometriosis. Being childless, having a history of pelvic infections, or having some kind of abnormality of the womb, have also been suggested as possible risk factors.

Professor Krina Zondervan, Principal Investigator at the Nuffield Department of Medicine at Oxford University, says:

> We know very little about the causes of endometriosis, which is typical of this complex disease. I became interested in the subject after studying chronic pelvic pain, as of course endometriosis is one of the causes. Until very recently research into the subject has been lagging behind. When I began working on it 15 or more years ago, most people didn't even know what it was! There is more awareness now and more information out there. Some genes linked to the condition have now been identified, but the influence of dietary or environmental factors is still not known. The animal studies in the 1990s suggested that being exposed to large quantities of dioxins could cause endometriosis in monkeys. Back in the 1970s there was an accident at a chemical plant in Italy and dioxins were released into the atmosphere. The affected areas were studied to see if reproductive disorders, including cancer and endometriosis, had developed in local women but any strong effect was ruled out and there hasn't been any similar research since.

Professor Zondervan's most recent research is into possible genetic causes of endometriosis (see Chapter 10). Her team is also looking at samples of endometrial tissue donated by volunteers to discover whether there are differences in what she describes as the 'stickiness' of cells – the ability of cells to adhere easily to other organs in the body outside the womb – between the endometrial tissue samples and other, normal, cells.

## Alternative theories

Mollie Hunton, a retired GP and qualified homoeopath from the West Midlands, agrees that endometriosis is likely to be multifactorial, or to have a combination of causes, but believes the main problem is that some women's immune systems are not equipped to deal with retrograde menstruation. She says:

> There are three exits from the womb – one is the cervix and the other two are the Fallopian tubes. When a woman is menstruating, the blood and endometrial cells are shed, and if the womb is not working as smoothly as it should, it pumps the blood and endometrium into the Fallopian tubes as well as the cervix. It's these uterine spasms which cause period cramps. As long as the woman's immune system is working well, this blood will be dealt with in the peritoneal cavity and will be re-absorbed without any problem. The evidence is all there. We know this retrograde menstruation happens to many women, and those with healthy immune systems can deal with it, while those who have a problem with their immune systems develop endometriosis.
>
> The health of the immune system has a lot to do with individual diets, lifestyles, and things like the over-use of antibiotics, which can strip the gut of its natural and friendly bacteria. It is the brain which switches a woman's immune system on or off and anything like a nasty shock, a bereavement or a period of stress can affect that. Then, if she has a damaged immune system, and possibly a genetic susceptibility to endometriosis as well, the condition will develop. The same situation in a different woman, who perhaps might have a genetic susceptibility to arthritis or multiple sclerosis, would lead to the development of those conditions instead. Modern medicine hasn't really put any of the apparent causes together, but if you do, and consider the whole

patient while looking at the bigger picture, then it becomes obvious.

Considering the whole person – in other words, treating women with endometriosis holistically – does seem to offer plenty of clues to the causes of endometriosis. We shall be looking at complementary therapies in detail in Chapter 9.

Hananja Brice-Ytsma is a medical herbalist who, after training in natural medicine in Holland, came to England and studied for a master's degree in women's health before lecturing at Middlesex University and treating those with the condition. She says:

> Women with endometriosis were referred to me by gynaecologists at the Whittington Hospital. I always took a very detailed medical history so that I got a full picture of what was going on for each woman, even though pain was the most important symptom they were dealing with. Endometriosis is known to be multifactorial and before I treated a woman I needed to know why it had occurred in this particular woman at this particular time. Contributory factors include oestrogen dominance, as tissue growth is dependent on oestrogen. The excess could just be too much oestrogen produced, or perhaps a deficiency of progesterone, the other main female hormone. Oestrogen dominance could be the result of liver weakness – the liver not working well – or the lymph drainage systems not working well. It's also important to look at digestion – does the woman have the wrong kind of gut flora? Is her bowel working properly? Does she suffer from nausea, bloating or constipation? A weakness in any of her body systems could be causing endometriosis to develop in an individual woman. Environmental factors could play a part too: we need to look at the use of pesticides and plastics. And there may be a genetic element. The fact that most women get retrograde menstruation but not all of them develop endometriosis suggests that there could be a weakness in the immune system for some, so they might need anti-inflammatories to help their white blood cells do their job in fighting infection.

# 4

# Getting a diagnosis

### How long does it take to get a diagnosis?

One of the most striking things, when researching this book, was discovering how long it takes for women to obtain a definite diagnosis of endometriosis! Even though endometriosis is the second most common gynaecological condition, and so many women are affected, I kept hearing of waits of two, four, six or even seven years before women actually found out what was wrong with them. When women do get a definite name for their condition, it often comes as a relief. One woman commented:

> It took me ages to convince my GP that I wasn't just making a fuss about ordinary period pains. In the end I had to insist that I was referred to a gynaecologist rather than being fobbed off with yet more painkillers that didn't work. I must have tried them all. I kept turning up at my local Accident and Emergency department in the middle of the night, begging for pain relief and anti-sickness medication. I was given morphine, pethidine – I'm sure the hospital thought I was some kind of addict! In the end they gave me something called ASPAV which is a mixture of aspirin and an opioid drug. I could administer this at home, so that at last I could get some sleep and relief from the awful pain.

Delays in diagnosis are still an issue for many women and, while things have improved, the average time, in the UK, is now around seven to seven and a half years, although some US studies have still confirmed a gap of 11 years or more. This may be because girls and women expect pain with their periods and many are unaware that, although period pain is common, it is not normal to be so debilitated by your monthly cycle that you are unable to go to school or work. Women may have suffered for several years before they even think to go to their GP. Doctors in London conducting the 2011 Global Study of Women's Health, which was funded by the World

Endometriosis Research Foundation (WERF; see Useful addresses), suggested that a major difficulty is getting women to visit their family doctor in the first place.[2] In addition to seeing period pain as normal, this may be because women:

- soldier on, not wanting to make a fuss about a natural process, especially if their peers seem to be managing;
- may be too embarrassed to go;
- may not open up about their symptoms once at the doctor's;
- may fear their doctor won't take them seriously.

Once through the surgery door, however, matters may be further delayed by the fact that not every doctor is aware of the many different symptoms of endometriosis. Those who are may very well prescribe the contraceptive pill (which can be an effective way of controlling the pain) rather than referring women to a gynaecologist for further investigations. Also, as we've seen, differential diagnosis is very common in endometriosis, IBS being one common misdiagnosis (see below). Researchers from the Global Study of Women's Health found that women are most commonly referred to a gastroenterologist, among other clinical specialists, before seeing a gynaecologist. This all means that diagnosis can take a long time.

However, it's important not to assume that your GP won't understand, or will just fob you off with painkillers. It is really helpful, as we have already said, to arm yourself with as much information as possible in the form of a pain diary and a symptom diary so that you are able to make it absolutely clear to the medical professionals that this is a period-related problem and that it is having a serious effect on your everyday life. In particular, check out the key symptoms of endometriosis (see page 9) and be very clear about which ones are affecting your life.

## Cathy

Cathy, who is 25 years old and is now expecting her first baby, says:

> I felt very frustrated when I eventually got a diagnosis and was told that treatment was possible. I started my periods rather young and always had an awful time. The pain was so excruciating that I had to miss school, but when I went to the doctor he said it was just one of those things. I was prescribed mefenamic acid – which did help – but

there was never any suggestion that the pain was anything but natural for me.

When I started work and was doubled up with pain once a month, my boss gave me a really hard time and I eventually had to leave. Naturally, I believed what the doctor had told me. How was I to know different? Even my honeymoon was a nightmare with leaking and flooding. My husband was very sympathetic but that was when I realized that what was happening to me was not normal. I was only diagnosed in the autumn of 2013 when we had been trying for a baby and nothing was happening. They thought I might have a blocked Fallopian tube but when I had a laparoscopy they found it was endometriosis. I had never heard of it but started investigating and found I'd had all the symptoms – pain, heavy bleeding, tiredness, constant urinary infections because the lesions were near my bladder. I really should have been diagnosed earlier.

## Diagnosing endometriosis

Once you get your appointment, you will be asked again to go into detail about your periods – when you started, if you have always had such severe pain, how heavy they are, how long they last – and about your other symptoms; for example, pain during or after sex, or when you use the loo. You may be given an internal examination at this point.

### Ultrasound

Ultrasound doesn't diagnose endometriosis itself, but does enable doctors to identify any cysts in your ovaries which may be caused by endometriosis. It can also be used to look for lesions in other areas, as well as whether your organs are stuck together by endometrial tissue. This is quite painless – a technician simply moves the ultrasound scanner across your pelvic area, and high frequency sound-waves are used to create an image on a screen.

### Laparoscopy

There are ongoing projects trying to devise a blood or urine test for endometriosis. Meanwhile, however, laparoscopy is often the gold standard (best possible test) in diagnosing endometriosis, although in practice ultrasound is often used first. It is also possible to try the pill and see if symptoms improve, before laparoscopy is used to get a definite diagnosis.

Laparoscopy is carried out under a general anaesthetic. A tiny cut is made beneath your navel and a viewing tube with a light, or laparoscope, is gently inserted into your pelvic area, enabling the doctor to see what is actually there. This might include endometrial nodules, lesions or cysts. Sometimes a biopsy (a small sample of tissue) is taken for further analysis, or obvious endometriosis might be removed straight away (see pages 34–5 for more details).

### A multi-disciplinary team

Consultant gynaecologist Bini Ajay of Spire St Anthony's Hospital says:

> Usually, diagnosis and treatment are done at the same time. However, some women may have very severe endometriosis which needs expert surgery by a multi-disciplinary team which may include, as well as a gynaecologist, a urologist and/or a colo-rectal surgeon. Their skills may be needed if the woman's bladder, ureter or bowel is affected by the endometriosis. If this is the case, a woman might also need medical and psychological preparation before the surgery can be performed, in case there are complications such as bowel surgery which may create the need for a colostomy bag afterwards.

## Is it endometriosis? Ruling out other conditions

One of the difficulties associated with diagnosis is that endometriosis mimics many conditions. These include Crohn's disease, cysts, diverticulitis, irritable bowel syndrome, pelvic inflammatory disease, ulcerative colitis, fibroids, even bowel and ovarian cancer. Given that women with endometriosis have a range of different symptoms, it's not hard to understand why other conditions may be suspected. Of course it is possible that, if you are unlucky, you are affected by one of these other conditions as well as your endometriosis. Other conditions include the following:

- *adenomyosis* produces pain and heavy and prolonged bleeding.

This condition, which used to be known as endometriosis interna, occurs when endometrial cells appear within the tissues in the uterine (womb) muscles, rather than elsewhere in the body. Just as in endometriosis, monthly hormonal changes cause them to swell up, leading to pain, heavy bleeding, and sometimes a feeling of heaviness as they press on the bladder or bowel. Bloating and fatigue can also be symptoms. You can learn more from a website <www.adenomyosisadviceassociation. org> (see Useful addresses), which was founded by a woman who battled it for years and had trouble getting any answers.

- *interstitial cystitis or bladder pain syndrome* can also be confused with endometriosis. One of its main symptoms is pain in the pelvic area, together with needing to urinate more often or very urgently. The pain may get worse around period time, which is why the confusion occurs. The cause isn't known but treatments range from self-help (pelvic exercises, giving up smoking) to medication.
- *adhesions* can cause pelvic pain in some women and means that the organs in the pelvic area get stuck together. Sometimes this is the result of endometriosis, but it can also happen when scars form after abdominal surgery (for instance, surgery for appendicitis), or if there is an injury to the area, or some kind of infection. Normal healthy organs are wrapped in a clear membrane called the peritoneum, and when this becomes inflamed it can cause pain and also bowel or bladder problems.
- *ovarian cysts* are very common and often appear for no apparent reason; they can disappear by themselves as well. Cysts can range in size from a pea to a melon, and most don't cause any symptoms unless they are very large, rupture or split, or they block the blood supply to the ovaries. In that case you might experience pelvic pain, a feeling of fullness and bloating, bowel problems, dizziness and extreme fatigue. Larger cysts may be surgically removed.
- *pelvic inflammatory disease* (PID) is a bacterial infection which spreads from the vagina to the rest of the genital tract including the womb, ovaries and Fallopian tubes. It can be caused by a sexually transmitted infection, or complications after a surgical operation, the insertion of an inter-uterine contraceptive device,

## Ovarian cancer

Persistent pelvic pain and bloating, a swollen abdomen and irregular bleeding after the menopause should always be checked out by your doctor. As with all forms of cancer, the earlier you are diagnosed and treated, the better the outcome, but ovarian cancer produces few symptoms in its early stages. In early ovarian cancer, when the disease is confined to the ovary, cure rates are approximately 70–90 per cent. Unfortunately, more than 70 per cent of women with ovarian cancer are diagnosed with advanced-stage disease, when the survival rate is only 20–30 per cent.

One study has come up with three hallmark symptoms of ovarian cancer in its early stages:

- abdominal and/or pelvic pain;
- feeling full quickly and/or being unable to eat normally;
- abdominal bloating and/or increased abdomen size.

The study, by researchers at Fred Hutchinson Cancer Research Center, Seattle and published online in the *Open Journal of Obstetrics and Gynecology*, is designed to be part of women's routine medical screening.[3] However, because such symptoms could be attributable to a wide range of causes, women should ask themselves if they are new, frequent, or continual in the past year and, if so, should talk to their doctor, according to lead researcher Dr M. Robyn Anderson of the University of Washington. Previous research by Andersen and colleagues found that some 60 per cent of women with early-stage ovarian cancer and 80 per cent of women with advanced disease report symptoms that follow this distinctive pattern at the time of diagnosis.

In the UK, consultant gynaecologist Bini Ajay, of Spire St Anthony's Hospital, suggests that one good way to remember the symptoms is through the acronym BEAT:

- B – bloating that is persistent;
- E – eating less and feeling fuller;
- A – abdominal pain;
- T – trouble with your bladder and bowels.

Dr Ajay advises paying attention to new and troublesome symptoms and never to assume that changes are due to age or diet.

or can occur after a miscarriage or abortion. It's more common in younger women and can cause the familiar symptoms of pelvic pain, pain during sex, irregular bleeding and bleeding after sex. PID is usually treated with antibiotics.

- *fibroids* are non-cancerous growths in the womb, which can vary in size from an apple pip to a grapefruit, or even larger in some cases. They are even more common than endometriosis, affecting as many as one in four women over the course of a lifetime. Like the other conditions described, they can cause similar symptoms of pain and heavy or prolonged periods. Fibroids seem to be more common in bigger women – those weighing more than 11 stone – and in those of African Caribbean heritage. Fibroids tend to shrink after the menopause and those that cause problems can be removed by surgery.

- *cystitis* – inflammation of the bladder – can also be a cause of pelvic pain. Most women have occasional cystitis; some women often get it. It can be treated with home remedies such as drinking plenty of water and/or cranberry juice, and taking simple painkillers or OTC medicines. Sometimes antibiotics are prescribed.

- *irritable bowel syndrome (IBS)* It isn't easy to distinguish pelvic pain involving the reproductive organs from similar pain caused by a disorder of the digestive tract. As a result of this, many women who see their GP and complain, rather vaguely, of stomach pain are diagnosed with IBS, which can produce quite similar symptoms to endometriosis. Irritable bowel syndrome is one of the most common digestive disorders in the Western world. It is described as a functional disorder, which means that your bowel doesn't process food as efficiently or as painlessly as it should. Instead, those affected by IBS have lower abdominal pain and bouts of either constipation or diarrhoea, or both. Bloating, fatigue and painful periods can also be symptoms. The causes of IBS are not really known although increased gut sensitivity, stress and an intolerance to particular foods have all been suggested. If IBS is a problem for you, you can get help and support in managing it from the IBS Network (see Useful addresses).

- *Crohn's disease and ulcerative colitis* are both inflammatory bowel disorders which can cause intermittent symptoms of pain and bowel upsets. In Crohn's, ulceration and scarring appear on the walls of the small intestine and elsewhere in the digestive tract. In ulcerative colitis it is the colon or large intestine which is affected, and the symptoms are very similar. Medication and/or a change in diet can help, with surgery as an option if these are not effective. Contact Crohn's and Colitis UK for more information (see Useful addresses).

- *diverticulitis*, a condition in which small, inflamed pouches appear on the bowel walls, is another condition which can cause pain, fatigue and bowel problems. It's more common in older people but may appear at any age. Medication and, if necessary, surgery can help. If you discover or suspect that a digestive disorder might be causing your symptoms you can find out more from Core, the Digestive Disorders Foundation (see Useful addresses).

With so many other conditions mimicking the symptoms caused by endometriosis, it becomes easier to see why endometriosis is difficult to spot without a full investigation. The more information you can give your GP about exactly what type of pain you have, where it is, how long you've had it and whether it seems to be related to your monthly cycle, the more clues he or she will have as to where to send you for further investigations.

## Ceri

Ceri had to wait 20 years before she was given a diagnosis of endometriosis.

> I was told I might have ovarian cysts, even though I had had very heavy, painful periods since I was 14. The pain was agonizing and I munched painkillers like sweets. My job as a sales consultant involved face-to-face-contact with the general public and half the time I would be doubled over in agony. I felt as if I'd been stabbed in the stomach.
>
> I think the answer is to find the right doctor. I changed several times until I found someone who actually said we needed to take a deeper look at what was happening. Credit where it's due, once things started moving I was soon referred to a specialist surgeon. The endometriosis was all over my ovaries and Fallopian tubes but hadn't spread outside the pelvic area, and it was removed with laser surgery. I suspect that he missed a bit because I still have some nagging pain. I have a Mirena coil, which really helps. It's hard to believe that no-one mentioned

endometriosis to me before – perhaps it was because I'd had the same symptoms since I was a teenager?

## Mina

Mina, 29, was diagnosed with adenomyosis three years ago, after having problem periods ever since she was 11.

My womb has ruled my life! When I was a teenager I had terrible migraines, vomiting, and just wanted to curl up in bed every month. I tried the pill, the mini-pill, Depo-Provera and an IUD but nothing seemed to help. Eventually, the condition was diagnosed with an MRI scan. Adenomyosis advances quite quickly and before I met my husband I begged for a hysterectomy because I thought it would get rid of the problem once and for all. Once I was married we began trying for a family but the fertility drugs I was prescribed made me put on weight, feel sick and lethargic and have awful mood swings. My husband got fed up with having to have sex on schedule too. After a fourth round of the drugs I did become pregnant with twins, but sadly I lost the babies at three and seven weeks. We were only entitled to one round of fertility treatment so we are now coming to terms with not being able to have a family.

I'm still wondering about having a hysterectomy. I'm young, I want to be able to enjoy my life. In the meantime I try to stay healthy. I go to the gym, I run and cycle and walk as much as I can which helps me not to feel depressed. I'm quite strict about diet too – no caffeine, no alcohol and of course no smoking. I also avoid anything that has a bloating effect, like fizzy drinks, white bread and pasta. I don't want my life to revolve around my adenomyosis any longer!

# 5

# Treatment

Because every woman's symptoms – and circumstances – are different, a variety of ways of managing endometriosis and easing the symptoms will be suggested. You'll need to discuss with both your GP and your gynaecologist exactly what is best for you. Depending on the exact nature of your symptoms, other specialists might also be involved in your treatment so that you are seeing a multi-disciplinary team. This could include experts in pain management, a urologist if the adhesions affect your bladder area, and a colo-rectal specialist if your bowel is affected. The treatment of endometriosis has several different aims:

- to offer some relief from the most painful symptoms and enable you to live a normal or near-normal life;
- to slow the growth of endometrial tissue so that endometriosis does not get any worse;
- to improve your chances of conceiving either right now, or in the future, depending on your age and future plans;
- to prevent the disease returning at a later date.

## To treat or not to treat?

Some women with very mild symptoms prefer to cope without treatment, especially if they are already nearing the menopause when their bodies are producing less oestrogen and symptoms may be becoming less severe. Some researchers have even claimed that symptoms will improve, even without any treatment. You might prefer not to take the chance, though! Pregnancy and breastfeeding do normally have an effect as while you are not ovulating or having periods, there's less chance of severe pelvic pain. Clearly, though, this is not an option for many women in today's world, although it could be a clue as to why endometriosis seems more common these days.

Few women in the Western world spend most of their adult lives either pregnant or as nursing mothers, as was the case in the past.

According to Endometriosis UK, some women even refuse pain-killers on the grounds that all these do is mask the pain, rather than getting to the root of the problem. However, they point out that choosing to do this, and remaining in pain, can pose a risk of developing neuropathic pain, where nerves send pain messages to the brain even when there is no specific injury or tissue damage to cause it.

## Medication

Painkilling medication is the first line of defence and can range from everyday painkillers like paracetamol and others which you can buy over the counter, to stronger drugs which are prescription-only. Painkillers act against the swelling and inflammation caused by endometriosis. It can help to begin a course of medication a few days before your period is expected – though, of course, if you're one of the unlucky women who have constant pain, or mid-cycle pain, that can be more difficult to plan. Paracetamol can help with milder pain and has few unwanted side effects in most women. Non-steroidal anti-inflammatories (NSAIDs), such as ibuprofen and mefenamic acid (Ponstan), work by blocking the production of prostaglandins, which are part of the body's naturally occurring response to injury, damage or disease. That's why it's important to begin taking a course of them before your body starts to produce these chemicals. However, you need to be aware that NSAIDs are not recommended for women with a history of stomach problems such as ulcers. Also, the NSAID Voltarol (diclofenac) is no longer recommended due to recent evidence of increased risk of heart attacks, and naproxen is used instead, usually with a stomach protectant such as omeprazole to prevent gastrointestinal damage. In addition, anti-inflammatory drugs such as ibuprofen and naproxen are contraindicated in those with other underlying health conditions, such as diabetes and kidney disease.

Endometriosis pain can also be treated with tricyclic anti-depressants such as amitriptyline, which, in addition to treating depression, have been found to have an effect on the nervous system by stopping pain messages from reaching the brain.

### Dealing with pain

TENS machines – the initials stand for TransCutaneous Electrical
Nerve Stimulation – seem to be effective in controlling pain for some
people. They are small, battery-operated devices that you wear. When
switched on, a small electrical impulse, which you feel as a tingle
or tickle, can block or reduce any pain signals, and this impulse,
also, apparently stimulates the production of endorphins, the body's
natural painkillers. You can buy TENS machines over the counter but
it's best to get advice from your doctor or physiotherapist about the
best and safest way to use them. They aren't, for example, suitable
for pregnant women, unless you are using them for pain relief during
labour, or anyone with a heart problem.

Some hospitals have a pain clinic where people can be taught
how to manage chronic pain. It's always worth asking if there is such
a clinic in your area. There are about 300 in the UK and you can find
out your nearest by looking at the British Pain Society website (see
Useful addresses). You have to be referred by your GP or consultant,
and what the clinics offer can vary. Many have teams of staff from
different medical disciplines – as well as doctors and nurses there
may be physiotherapists, occupational therapists and psychologists.
A variety of treatments may be offered including acupuncture and
hypnotherapy. Pain management techniques may also be taught.

## Hormonal treatments

Endometriosis is a hormone-related condition, in that the endometrial cells respond to fluctuating hormone levels every month
no matter where they are in the body. Women often find that if
they become pregnant, or as they approach the menopause, the
changing levels of the main female hormone oestrogen mean that
symptoms change, become less troublesome, and may even disappear altogether.

Hormone treatments for endometriosis interfere with the
normal process of oestrogen production, in the hope of allevi-
ating symptoms. It can help if you understand exactly how the
oestrogen-producing process actually works. It begins when the
brain produces a special hormone called GnRH or gonadotrophin-
releasing hormone. This travels to the pituitary gland (next to the

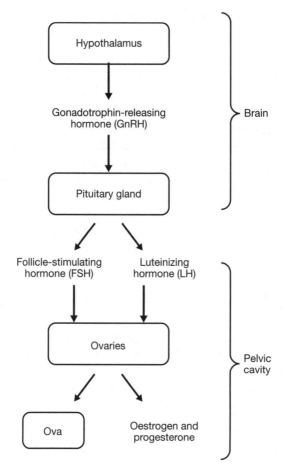

**Figure 3 The oestrogen-producing process**

brain) enabling it to produce gonadotrophins in its turn. When these are released into your bloodstream, they stimulate your ovaries to produce the female hormone oestrogen (Figure 3).

Without oestrogen, endometrial tissue can be reduced (although it's important to be aware that reducing oestrogen may not have any effect on adhesions in the pelvic organs).

There are several different ways of treating endometriosis with hormones. Finding the right one for you might involve trying different approaches and will depend on the severity of your symptoms and the possible side effects produced by the treatment. For example, you might be offered:

- *the combined pill or a contraceptive patch.* The combined pill or patch contains a combination of oestrogen and progestogen and may relieve milder symptoms. Because the pill stops ovulation – the release of an egg each month – it should mean that your periods will become lighter and less painful. It's safe to take the pill continuously without a break, and if you find that a particular pill causes unwanted side effects – the most common being nausea, breast tenderness, irregular bleeding, bloating and weight gain – there are several different brands that you can try until you find one that suits you. Some gynaecologists prefer to prescribe the progestogen-only or mini-pill to women for whom the combined pill isn't suitable – for example those who are smokers, have high blood pressure or have had a deep-vein thrombosis.
- *a Mirena coil* (the IUS or intra-uterine contraceptive system). This is a T-shaped device which is fitted into your womb. It prevents the womb lining growing too quickly and makes it thinner. It may stop your periods altogether and will reduce any pain. You can leave the Mirena coil in for four or five years quite safely. It suits many women very well, although possible side effects may include irregular bleeding, breast tenderness and acne.

Megan, 39, has had a Mirena coil for six years and says it has changed her life. Megan is one of those women who was unaware that endometriosis was the cause of her gynaecological problems, the most troublesome of which was unbearably heavy periods.

> They had always been really heavy especially in the first couple of days. I had to change my tampon every 90 minutes or so which was awful especially if I was travelling. I experienced a few side effects after I had the coil fitted, like increased PMS and swollen breasts, but they weren't as much trouble as my periods had been. I understand that some women don't have periods at all when they have a Mirena coil but I still do, which is reassuring. I know women for whom it wasn't the right choice but it certainly worked for me.

It's important to remember that these three kinds of treatment – the pill, the patch and the Mirena coil – have a contraceptive effect, unlike other forms of hormone treatment. If you are planning to become pregnant in the near future, you should discuss with your GP whether these are appropriate treatments for you at this time.

**GnRH analogues** Other types of hormone treatment include GnRH analogues, such as triptorelin (trade name Gonapeptyl), buserelin, goserelin (trade name Zoladex), nafarelin, and leuprorelin (trade name Prostap). These are synthetic hormones which reduce oes- trogen production, producing a temporary, artificial menopause in the women who take them. The drugs are available in the form of a monthly injection and are usually prescribed for just six months at a time because it has been discovered that if women take them for any longer than that they can suffer from up to 20 per cent bone loss. Like most drugs they may have side effects, which are similar to the effects of a natural menopause – hot flushes, low libido and vaginal dryness. Because of this, some women are prescribed hormone replacement therapy (HRT) alongside the treatment. Although this might seem illogical – why take strong drugs to reduce the amount of oestrogen produced and then replace it? – the amount of oestrogen in HRT is very small and shouldn't be enough to cause problems.

**Progestogens** These are a synthetic form of the female hormone progesterone which works by preventing the womb lining from growing too quickly. They are usually taken in the form of tablets which you take from day 5 to day 26 of your menstrual cycle. Some women tolerate them well; other get side effects such as mood swings, bloating, irregular bleeding and weight gain.

**Other hormone treatments** such as danazol and Gestrinone are derivatives of the male hormone testosterone, which are used like GnRH analogues, to lower the levels of oestrogen being produced. Unwanted side effects, as well as those described above, may include increased hair growth and a deepening voice so these are being prescribed less often as better alternatives are available. If you are on danazol, there is evidence that exercise improves or reduces side effects.

**Aromatase inhibitors** are drugs which suppress the production of aromatase, an enzyme which is critical in the production of oestrogen. In the 1990s, researchers discovered that endometrial tissue outside the womb seemed to produce high levels of aromatase. Drugs which, until then, had been used to treat some women, especially older women, with breast cancer were tried, on an experimental basis, on women with endometriosis which had not responded to other treatments. The drugs involved were anastrozole (Arimidex) and letrozole (Femara). Although there have been no large-scale trials they seemed to be successful in controlling pain and to produce only mild side effects, such as hot flushes and loss of libido. It is also thought that long-term use of these drugs might lead to bone loss (osteoporosis) so, where they have been used, it has usually been in combination with other drugs, and calcium and Vitamin D supplements. Research and clinical trials only seem to have taken place outside the UK, however, and these drugs are not currently available here either privately or on the NHS.

**Visanne**   Another new drug, which is available for use in some parts of Europe and also Canada, has the brand name Visanne and is a kind of progestogen called dienogest. It's a long-term, oral treatment not unlike the progestogen-only or mini-pill. It has been widely studied abroad and appears to work by suppressing the effects of oestrogen (in the form of estradiol) on endometrial tissue, which reduces the pain. It is said to be well tolerated with side effects similar to other hormone treatments (nausea, headache, breast pain) which wear off once your body is used to it. There have already been campaigns in Australia and New Zealand to make this new treatment available. At the time of writing, NICE, the National Institute for Health and Care Excellence, which evaluates new drug and other treatments, has said that more research is needed before it can be licensed for the treatment of endometriosis here.

## Surgery

Surgery is another option to consider, particularly if medication has not worked very well for you. Again, it is a choice you can only make for yourself – in conjunction with your GP and consultant – and will depend on your age, medical history and circumstances.

For example, you won't want to consider a total hysterectomy if you are planning to start a family, or if you are hoping to add to your family.

## Laparoscopy

As well as being the technique used to diagnose your endometriosis, laparoscopy is also a form of surgical treatment. It is common and only minimally invasive, making very small incisions and leaving you with a tiny scar which soon fades. A laparoscope, a thin tube with a light source and a camera, is inserted into a small incision in the lower abdomen to show an image of the endometriosis, which is then relayed to a TV screen. Depending on where exactly it is, how extensive it is, and what type of endometriosis it is – adhesions, chocolate cysts, nodules, lesions – an array of delicate instruments will be used to apply heat, a laser, an electric current or a beam of helium gas to the endometrial tissue, which is either destroyed or cut out completely. Most surgeons have their own preferred method and instruments so you should ask the surgeon performing your operation exactly how it will be done – if you want to know!

You will be given a general anaesthetic for this procedure, which is often done on an outpatient basis, although you may have to spend one night in hospital. Recovery time is faster than for more extensive surgery and can be anything from one day to a couple of weeks. The only complications occur if some of the endometrial tissue is left behind, in which case the symptoms may recur.

Caroline Overton is a consultant gynaecologist at St Michael's University Hospital in Bristol. She is also Lead for the University Hospitals Bristol NHS Foundation Trust Endometriosis Centre and a member of Endometriosis UK's Medical Advisory Panel. She says:

> It's usually possible to have this surgery as a day case, but what is carried out at the time of the operation depends on where the endometriosis is, and what has been agreed with you beforehand. Your surgeon will advise you on how long you will need off work afterwards. I would advise women to book at least two weeks off, so that they can have the time they need to recover. You can go home after the operation as soon as you can walk, eat and drink, pass urine, and are comfortable with oral painkillers.

The general assumption is that because the cuts are small, this is only minor surgery. However, it is the surgery inside that decides whether an operation is major or minor, and it is possible to carry out major surgery through keyhole cuts. Your stomach will feel tender because of the cuts that have been made. These make you feel as though you have done too many sit-ups, and the effect of the surgery inside can feel like period pains, or a flare-up of the endometriosis. This is because the areas of endometriosis have been excised (cut out) or diathermied (burned away) or lasered. As soon as you go home, it is safe for you to walk up stairs, have a shower or bath, and lift a kettle or one small bag of shopping. You should expect to feel very tired and it is normal to need a rest after routine jobs that you would have done without even thinking about. Your normal energy will return as you recover.

Your tummy muscles will feel sore, and to make getting out of bed more comfortable it's better to roll onto your side, drop your feet onto the floor, and come up sideways. It's fine to have a bath but go for a quick dip rather than a long soak while the cuts are still covered with plasters. Trapped wind can be unexpectedly painful and peppermint tea can help. The operation can affect your appetite, so make sure you have plenty of easy to digest and quick to prepare food in the house. Soup is ideal. It's a myth that surgery will make you put on weight, but while you are less active you won't need the same amount of calories that you usually eat.

Your surgeon will guide you on when you should be ready to go back to work. Most women are ready to go back two to six weeks after their operation. You can go back to driving as soon as you have come off the stronger painkillers, as these can make you feel drowsy. You need to be able to sit comfortably in the driving seat, wear the seat belt, turn to look in the mirrors, and make an emergency stop. I would advise you to practise these manoeuvres in a stationary car before you decide that you can go out on the road. You should also check with your car insurance as they may have specific requirements.

Megan was only recently diagnosed with endometriosis after laparoscopy to remove a cyst. She says:

My gynaecologist told me there was a risk I might have to have more complex surgery, depending on what they found, so I was very relieved to wake up and find out that keyhole surgery had been used. I had a few days off work and recovered really quickly. I was told I had endometriosis around my bladder and affecting my left Fallopian tube but they removed as much as possible at the same time.

## Laparotomy

Laparotomy is a slightly more complex and invasive operation which is used when the endometriosis is more severe, or where it has caused the organs in the pelvic cavity to fuse together. A wide cut along the bikini line has to be made in order to remove the endometrial tissue and, as this is a more serious operation, recovery will be slower.

## Hysterectomy

The removal of the womb, sometimes with the ovaries and Fallopian tubes as well, can be an option for women whose families are complete and for whom other kinds of treatment just haven't worked. It is, however, a major operation. Your operation may be:

- a total hysterectomy, where your womb and cervix are removed;
- a sub-total hysterectomy, where your womb, but not your cervix, is removed;
- a total hysterectomy with bilateral salpingo-oophorectomy, where your womb, cervix, Fallopian tubes and ovaries are removed;
- a radical hysterectomy, where your womb, cervix, Fallopian tubes, ovaries, part of your vagina, lymph glands and fatty tissue are removed.

Consultant gynaecologist Bini Ajay says:

> The treatments chosen for an individual will depend on her symptoms and the severity of the endometriosis, whether the choice is progestogen treatment, the Mirena coil, diathermy – which is the use of a high frequency electric current to generate deep heat in body tissues – or a total hysterectomy with bilateral salpingo-oophorectomy, which can either be done by keyhole or open surgery.

As hysterectomy is classed as major surgery you are likely to be in hospital for about five days and complete recovery could take six to eight weeks. The fitter you are, the quicker your recovery is likely to be. Your consultant can answer any questions you may have about the operation and its aftermath, or you can find out more from the Hysterectomy Association website (see Useful addresses). Bear in mind that if your ovaries are not removed, it is more likely that the symptoms of endometriosis may recur. Hysterectomy is only a cure for endometriosis if all the affected organs are removed. If the lesions have spread to other parts of the body, you might still have symptoms after your operation.

## Menopause

The average age for menopause in the UK is around 51. Whatever your age, if you have your ovaries removed you will go through the menopause straight after your operation. If one or both ovaries remain, you will reach your menopause within five years. It may be trouble-free or you may experience typical symptoms of hot flushes, mood swings and vaginal dryness. If you have a surgical menopause after a hysterectomy, you'll need to discuss with your GP and consultant whether you need to take hormone replacement therapy (HRT). Again this is very much an individual decision especially as there are several different kinds of HRT to be considered. Oestrogen-only types carry a slight risk of the endometriosis returning, and as you no longer have a womb, you will not need the protective effect of progestogen, another hormone which helps to protect against womb cancer.

## Women's experiences of treatment

Women's experiences of treatment vary tremendously. Most say that finding the right doctor is absolutely crucial.

### Alison

Alison has suffered from severe period pain and pain when she used the loo, ever since she was a teenager.

> I moved house several times and found that every gynaecologist I saw had his or her own ideas about what was the best treatment. Luckily, they discovered that the endometriosis was around my bladder and

bowel rather than my reproductive organs, so I had no trouble getting pregnant. The pain started again when my boys were small and I seem to have tried everything, including a GnRH analogue plus HRT, and hypnotherapy which helped to relieve the stress of feeling permanently ill! In the end I opted for a hysterectomy and it was the best decision I ever made. I can now live a normal life again – eat whatever I fancy, go away on holiday – without being crippled by pain.

## Ceri

Ceri, 39, says:

Even though I'd had problems ever since I hit puberty, it was years before I was offered any really helpful treatment. Once I found a sympathetic consultant who seemed to want to take a really good look, everything moved quite fast and I was operated on with a laser by a specialist surgeon.

## Amy

Amy is 32 and waiting to hear about her initial assisted conception appointment.

I think I have tried everything. I tried several different contraceptive pills at first, which worked for a time but then the heavy bleeding returned. My first laparoscopy revealed Stage II endometriosis. I was put on Zoladex for two sessions of six months each but it made me feel terrible with mood swings, crippling headaches and weight gain as well as bursting into tears at the slightest thing. When I had the next operation they found the endometriosis had increased to Stage IV and not shrunk at all. I lived with it for a few years and then had still more surgery where the endometriosis was excised rather than burned away with a laser, and that seemed to be more successful. I had regular operations all through my twenties and thanks to those and prescription painkillers there was only one day when I couldn't go into work. I have now been married for two years and because of my health problems my husband and I decided to try for a baby sooner rather than later.

# 6

# 'Will I be able to have children?'

For some women, a diagnosis of endometriosis only comes when they have been trying to conceive for some time and nothing is happening. Indeed, a common complaint is that endometriosis is often only viewed by the medical profession in terms of how it affects fertility, leaving its wider health implications ignored. It's also true that other factors affecting fertility must be taken into account if you have endometriosis – that is, don't be too quick to blame endometriosis for any delay in conceiving. The good news is that it is possible to conceive even if you have endometriosis.

### The myth that endometriosis means infertility

Too many women believe, or are led to believe, that endometriosis invariably equals infertility. This just isn't so. If you have been diagnosed, you shouldn't assume that your chances of having a family are zero. Unfortunately, there are no reliable statistics on what percentage of women with endometriosis have difficulties becoming pregnant. However, an estimated 60–70 per cent of women with endometriosis are fertile. Furthermore, about half the women who have difficulties becoming pregnant do eventually conceive with or without treatment. So, while endometriosis can be a factor in infertility, many women with endometriosis do have children.

A great deal depends on where exactly in your body, the endometrial lesions or 'chocolate cysts' are, and whether your reproductive organs (ovaries and Fallopian tubes) are more affected than your bowel or bladder. Fertility may also be affected by the severity of your condition, by other factors (see below) and, as applies to women without endometriosis, by your age. In medical terms, infertility is defined as not becoming pregnant after one year of regular intercourse. According to Endometriosis UK, it's important to remember that:

- if you have mild or medium endometriosis, you will probably have no problem getting pregnant;
- if your endometriosis is severe, it may have caused adhesions (scar tissue) to form around your reproductive organs and you are likely to have more problems conceiving;
- there is a link between endometriosis and infertility, but researchers have not yet managed to work out exactly what it is;
- conception is still possible, even if your endometriosis is severe.

## Other fertility problems

Fertility is a complex issue, and endometriosis is far from the only reason why approximately one in seven British couples have problems conceiving. The most significant reason of all is age. Fertility in healthy women tends to decline sharply after the age of 38 or so. Of course we all know women who have happy healthy babies in their 40s, but that is still a general rule and something women should bear in mind if they believe their lives would be incomplete without children of their own. Women aged 35–39 have about half the chance of conceiving of women aged 19–26. Other reasons why couples may find it difficult to conceive include:

- lack of regular ovulation (the release of a monthly egg into the Fallopian tubes);
- polycystic ovary syndrome, where harmless cysts, often under-developed egg sacs which never release an egg, develop in your ovaries;
- blocked Fallopian tubes so that the egg is unable to travel down into the womb.

In about a third of cases of infertility, it's the woman who has a problem. In another third, it's the man, who may be producing poor quality sperm. In another third, everything seems to be working normally but the diagnosis is unexplained infertility, which is, of course, distressing and frustrating for the couple concerned. If more than one risk factor – for example age, blocked tubes, low sperm count – is present, then your chances of conceiving naturally are reduced. Endometriosis, then, is just one of the possible reasons why a woman may not be able to conceive. That doesn't, however, mean there is no hope.

## How endometriosis affects fertility

We have already learned how endometriosis can affect any of the organs in the pelvic area and cause cysts, adhesions and scarring that can distort these important organs and make conception more difficult. Severe adhesions, forming scar tissue rather like cobwebs, may wrap around the ovaries and simply prevent the egg from passing down the Fallopian tubes and into the womb. There is also the point that some women with endometriosis find penetrative sex extremely painful, thus reducing chances of conception. If this is the case with you, do see your GP or go to a sexual health (genito-urinary medicine or GUM) clinic to discuss ways to make you more comfortable.

### Classification of Endometriosis Score

The American Fertility Society has produced a Classification of Endometriosis Score, based on considerations such as the part of the pelvic organs affected, the presence of ovarian cysts, the amount of scar tissue and the degree to which organs have stuck together, and divided endometriosis into:

- stage I – minimal
- stage II – mild
- stage III – moderate
- stage IV – severe (see Figure 4).

As we've already said, you can't assess how severe your endometriosis is by how severe your pain is. This classification is used to assess the impact on fertility, rather than classifying the endometriosis itself.

It's estimated that:

- of 100 women without endometriosis having regular sex for a year, 84 will get pregnant;
- of 100 women with minimal/mild endometriosis (stages I and II) having regular sex for a year, 75 will get pregnant;

Stage I, minimal

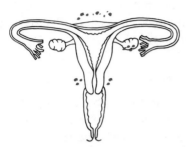

Endometriosis in
peritoneum and
right ovary

Stage II, mild

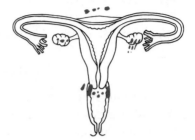

Endometriosis in
peritoneum, right
and left ovaries

Stage III, moderate

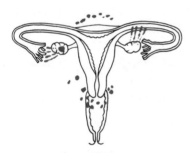

Endometriosis in
peritoneum, right and
left tubes and right
and left ovaries

Stage IV, severe

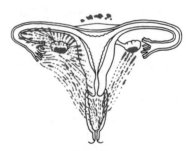

Endometriosis in
peritoneum, right
and left ovaries
and left tube

**Figure 4 Stages of endometriosis**

- of 100 women with moderate endometriosis (stage III) having regular sex for a year, 50 will get pregnant;
- of 100 women with severe endometriosis (stage IV) having regular sex for a year, 25 will get pregnant.

## Getting help

If you are trying to start a family and nothing is happening, you'll need a full series of investigations to discover exactly what the problems are – in other words, whether it is only the fact that you have endometriosis which is stopping you from conceiving, or whether there are other factors involved, either to do with your own health or your partner's.

Couples are usually advised to go to their GP if they have been trying for a baby without success for a year. However, if you (the female partner) are over 36, you should ask for an appointment without waiting for a year. Six months is sometimes suggested. If you have already been diagnosed with endometriosis – perhaps because you have had a lot of problems with your periods since you were a teenager – then you might not want to wait a year either, just in case conception is going to be difficult for you. It may also be helpful to contact the Infertility Network UK (see Useful addresses). This organization has a wide range of expertise on fertility issues and they also have a factsheet on endometriosis.

Megan, who is 39, was only recently diagnosed with endometriosis.

> When I discovered I had endometriosis I felt rather confused. My gynae-cologist told me that getting pregnant could help with my symptoms but that because my Fallopian tubes were affected I might have trouble conceiving. I am in a fairly new relationship and I know my age is against me. I have seen friends go down the assisted conception route and know how difficult it can be. I'm not sure that I want a family enough to go through that – but at this point I wouldn't want further surgery which would take that choice away from me.

If you are being treated for endometriosis, and you want to get pregnant now, it is very important to remember that all the current drugs used to treat endometriosis – apart from very simple pain-killers such as paracetamol – are not recommended for use during pregnancy in case they cause harm to the developing foetus. If you are planning to start a family, take advice from your GP or consultant about coming off your medication first.

If you want a baby one day, but not now, you should consider taking the combined contraceptive pill, which contains two hormones, oestrogen and progestogen. Because it prevents ovulation, it reduces pain, controls endometriosis symptoms, and may even help to slow the progress of the condition. Depending on your symptoms your doctor may suggest that you take it continuously, which means without the usual seven-day break. There are several different brands of pill you can try. They all contain different types of oestrogen and progestogen in slightly different doses, so it's likely you will be able to find one to suit you if you are troubled by side effects at first.

It appears that if you are taking medication for endometriosis, and come off the drugs in order to start a family, your chances of conceiving may not have been improved. It can take time for your fertility to return to normal. The female hormonal system is a delicately balanced thing. Some complementary practitioners believe that if you have used one of the types of hormonal contraception which suppresses your periods altogether, your body may 'forget' how to bleed regularly, which obviously reduces your chances of conceiving.

However, if you have surgical treatment – such as a laparoscopy or laparotomy (see Chapter 5) for endometriosis – a skilled surgical procedure will destroy the nodules, release any adhesions, and remove any cysts in your ovaries, and this does improve your chances of conceiving. If you have had an operation you should wait for a year and see if you become pregnant naturally, before exploring other options such as IVF (in-vitro fertilization).

Whether or not you have already been diagnosed with endometriosis, if you are having regular unprotected sex (that means every two or three days) and not conceiving, you will need to go through a number of fertility tests before you find out what exactly is wrong and what the best course of treatment might be in your particular circumstances. Fertility testing is without doubt a stressful experience and, as there is evidence that stress can affect your chances of conceiving, it's important that both you and your partner try to relax as much as possible. Severe stress can disrupt your ovulation cycle, reduce your partner's sperm count and also increase the number of abnormal sperm. We shall be looking at specific stress reduction techniques in Chapter 8. It's important at every stage of the investigations that you reduce other stress factors in both your lives as much as possible.

The aim of any investigations is to find out what factors are affecting your ability to conceive naturally – and, of course, endometriosis might be one of these. In addition, and before you are referred to a specialist, your GP will probably ask questions about:

- your age, as women's fertility begins to decline from their mid-thirties onward;
- your past medical history, including any pregnancies or miscarriages, or serious illnesses, such as cancer;
- your experience of sex. Please try not to be embarrassed, the doctors just want to know exactly what's happening. For example, if you're reluctant to have intercourse regularly because you find it painful, that will have a bearing on your chances of conceiving. It can also be helpful to calculate your most fertile time of the month – five days before ovulation and one day after – which means between days 10 and 17 if you have a regular 28-day cycle. Making love at this most fertile time can obviously improve your chances;
- the type of contraception you have been using – when you stop using contraception it can sometimes take a little time for your system to return to normal;
- your periods – are they regular, painful, excessively heavy? Do you pass a lot of clots of blood? Is there any bleeding or spotting between periods?
- any medication you are taking (prescribed or complementary);
- your lifestyle and your partner's, including things like how much you smoke or drink and how stressed you are. Smoking, for example, is a no-no if you are trying to conceive. Not only can it damage eggs, sperm and embryos but it also reduces the chances of success with IVF and increases your risk of miscarriage. Street drugs, of course, are likewise not to be recommended;
- your weight – women who are seriously over- or underweight sometimes have problems conceiving.

You may also be given a pelvic examination so that your GP can check for any possible infection, lumps and bumps or any pain in the pelvic area. Your partner will also be given a genital examination so that any problems can be picked up at this early stage. He will be asked for a sperm sample so that he can be checked for abnormalities.

If your GP suspects that endometriosis could be a factor, you could be referred for a laparoscopy at this point. There are other tests you could be offered as well, either through your GP surgery or in hospital.

## Further investigations

Other investigations include blood tests to:

- reveal whether or not you are experiencing problems with ovulation by measuring the levels of the hormone progesterone in a blood sample taken seven days before your period is due;
- check for rubella (German measles) which can be harmful in the first three months of pregnancy.

Urine tests:

- for women to reveal problems in ovulation by measuring the levels of luteinizing hormone in your urine. A blood test, taken during your period, can also reveal LH levels, as well as the levels of follicle-simulating hormone (FSH) and estradiol. The test might also identify a possible early menopause, which could affect your chances of conceiving.
- for men to check for the very common sexually transmitted infection chlamydia, which can also affect sperm function and male fertility.

Other tests:

- a vaginal swab with a cotton bud can be used to test for the presence of chlamydia, which can cause pelvic inflammatory disease and fertility problems. If present, chlamydia can be treated with a course of antibiotics;
- a cervical smear test might also be offered if you haven't had one recently;
- an ultrasound scan is sometimes used to check on the condition of your womb, ovaries and Fallopian tubes;

- an X-ray of your Fallopian tubes, known as an HSG or hysterosalpingogram, will reveal whether or not they are blocked;
- a full hormone profile could be offered to check for hormonal imbalances;
- follicle tracking via ultrasound can check whether your egg follicles and your eggs are developing properly;
- a hysteroscopy (a telescope with attached camera) may be used to check your womb for polyps or fibroids;
- a laparoscopy, as we have already seen, will show whether you have endometriosis, if this has not already been diagnosed.

## Fertility treatment

Fertility treatment does offer couples a chance of having their own babies, but it isn't an easy option, whether or not endometriosis is a factor. According to the Infertility Network, whether or not you are offered treatment on the NHS depends almost entirely on where you live – the so-called postcode lottery. At the time of writing, the most up-to-date guidelines from NICE (published in February 2013) stated that in England, women under 39 should be offered three cycles of IVF on the NHS, and women between 40 and 42, whose chances of conception are lower, one cycle. However these guidelines are not mandatory, so you could find that in your area there may be more restrictions. In Wales, women are entitled to two full cycles but there are long waiting lists. In Scotland, two or three cycles may be offered where there are 'reasonable expectations' of a live birth and the position was reviewed in early 2015.

However, the campaigning group Fertility Fairness (see Useful addresses) found that these guidelines were often not adhered to, and that the position was changing all the time depending on financial constraints. They found that only 38 clinical commissioning groups in NHS England actually offered three cycles, 61 offered two, and 110 offered couples just one – and they found that one area offered none at all. This can leave couples with no choice but to opt for private treatment which can cost £5000 or more per cycle.

If you are accepted for fertility treatment, it can be a gruelling process physically, as well as being emotionally stressful. Depending on the degree of endometriosis you have, and whether there are other factors involved, such as a partner's low sperm count, different processes can be involved. You will normally have to take a drug which stimulates your ovaries to produce more eggs. The drugs can be taken via a nasal spray which you use several times a day, or you can have a daily or monthly injection.

If you are a young woman with clear Fallopian tubes, who ovulates regularly, and your partner is producing healthy sperm, then these will be selected and inserted into your womb, via your cervix, using a very thin plastic tube at a carefully calculated time so that egg and sperm have the best chance of meeting up. This process is known as ovulation induction with intra-uterine insemination.

IVF can be used for women who have severe endometriosis, even if their Fallopian tubes are blocked by adhesions. The first step is ovarian stimulation. Naturally, your ovaries produce one egg every month, and it is possible for this one egg to be mixed with your partner's sperm and for the resulting embryo to be replaced in your uterus. However, success rates if this is done are not very high, so it's usual for women to be treated with drugs called gonadotrophins which lead the ovaries to produce more eggs.

The next stage – egg recovery – is carefully timed and takes place under sedation or a general anaesthetic. A number of eggs may be harvested and placed in a laboratory dish where they are mixed with your partner's sperm. Sometimes, a technique called ICSI – intracytoplasmic sperm injection – is used, in which one especially healthy and mobile sperm is selected and injected directly into an egg. Then, once the resulting embryo has developed into what is called a blastocyte, which takes a few days, it will be replaced into your womb. To avoid the possibility of multiple pregnancies, usually only one or two embryos are used: the others can be stored if you wish. You may also be treated with the hormone progesterone (Cyclogest, Gestone, Crinone) which helps to thicken the lining of the womb in order to maintain the pregnancy – either in the form of a vaginal suppository, a pill, a gel or an injection.

Like all drugs, hormone treatments such as these can have side effects, which can range from stomach pains to hot flushes, mood swings, tender breasts, insomnia, weight gain, spots, dizziness and vaginal dryness. Not everyone gets these, but it's important to report them to your doctor or clinic if they are really troublesome.

Fertility treatment is, of course, always tailored to individual circumstances so there may be other factors to consider which are not related to your endometriosis. You may need or want to have your embryos screened for any genetic problems. You may need donated eggs or sperm. You may even consider surrogacy – when another woman carries your child for you – with all its emotional, financial and legal implications. Commercial surrogacy – paying a woman to have a child for you – is illegal in the UK, though you are allowed to pay reasonable expenses. The Human Fertilisation and Embryology Authority (HFEA; see Useful addresses) recommends that anyone considering this should take legal advice first.

Assisted conception, however it happens, can never be an easy option, particularly as there is no guarantee that it will result in a pregnancy and a healthy baby. The HFEA says that success rates, on average, range from 32.2 per cent for women under 35 to just 5 per cent for women aged 43–44. They have a booklet called *Getting Started – your guide to infertility treatment* available from their website <www.hfea.gov.uk>.

## Miranda

I was 39 and newly married when we realized getting pregnant was not going to be easy. My GP, who had been a late mum herself, was very sympathetic and referred me to the nearest IVF clinic. I found the whole process deeply unpleasant. Basically, IVF takes over your whole menstrual cycle. You are injected with lots of drugs so that your ovaries produce more eggs. I felt bloated and as if I had permanent PMS – weepy and irrational.

I had to go to the hospital at unpredictable intervals to have my hormone levels checked and then had egg harvesting under sedation. I think they harvested about four. Then we were told that John's sperm sample wasn't up to scratch and only one egg fertilized naturally. I didn't become pregnant and we both felt awful. I felt old and past it and John felt that it was his fault. It took all the spontaneity out of our love life and the procedures felt totally unnatural.

The consultant told us that if we wanted another go, I would need more drugs and our chances of a pregnancy at my age were less than 5 per cent. I had some counselling but really, the decision was made and we decided not to try again. The truth is, even today, women's fertility does decline in their late thirties and endometriosis means the odds are against you. I wouldn't blame anyone for keeping on trying but I sometimes wonder if knowing there is even a 5 per cent chance just prolongs the misery of infertility.

## Cathy

Cathy, 25, is one of the lucky ones. Even though she had had symptoms ever since her periods started, she wasn't diagnosed until she had been married and trying to start a family for five years. In late 2013 she had a laparoscopy which revealed that she had endometriosis.

> I'd never heard of it even though I had all the classic symptoms, from heavy bleeding and clots to extreme tiredness. The surgery revealed that I had deep scar tissue near my bladder, which might explain all the urinary tract infections I had had!
>
> I had another operation a few months later to burn away the endometriosis and was told to continue to try to conceive naturally for six months before thinking about assisted conception. After the operation I felt so much better, almost like a new person. I did some research on the internet and learned more about the condition, including the fact that it might come back, even though I had been told I had a good chance of becoming pregnant. The months passed and nothing happened . . . until, at Month Six, I didn't get my period and a test revealed I was pregnant! We felt very lucky and very blessed when our son was born in February 2015.

## Marie

Marie, 34, had been seeing her GP for severe period pains ever since she was a teenager and was offered nothing more than painkillers and a hot-water bottle until she changed GPs in 2005.

> I knew what was happening to me every month wasn't right and I asked for a referral to a gynaecologist. At last I found someone who listened and understood. I had a laparoscopy and they found a lot of endometriosis around my ovaries and bowel which was removed. No-one mentioned fertility at that stage. The pain kept coming back and I had further operations to remove the lesions.
>
> In 2007 I got married and we began trying for a family. Nothing happened. We had all the tests and eventually I saw a consultant in London. He told me that in some women with endometriosis, the little filaments in the Fallopian tubes don't work properly so the egg doesn't pass down the tube. In others, it's the fluid around the cervix that prevents the

sperm getting to the womb. In both those cases the sperm and egg just never meet up.

We went straight for IVF. It was daunting to begin with. You have to be really motivated to put up with the idea of daily injections. The increase in hormone levels gave me PMT as well. It was a real test of our marriage – which we passed I'm glad to say! Nine eggs were retrieved, four fertilized, and two were put back. Two weeks later I did a test and found that I was pregnant. I was then given a progesterone pessary to thicken the womb lining so the embryo would have a better chance to implant. Then we had the six-week wait for the first scan when we heard the heartbeat. I sometimes wonder how we got through it.

The pregnancy was horrendous. Physically I felt well, with no pain, but I was so afraid something would go wrong that I couldn't relax and enjoy it. Our son was born by emergency C-section in 2011, weighing nine pounds nine ounces. It wasn't a straightforward birth as there were endometriosis nodules on the placenta, which burst, and I lost three pints of blood. But he was healthy and strong and still is.

I have been all right without medication for more than three years now. I do have some pain and tiredness but I just thank my lucky stars that we have our son. I would like to give him a brother or sister but we would have to pay privately for more IVF and it's not an option at the moment. We know how fortunate we are.

## Beth

Beth and her husband were diagnosed with unexplained infertility after two years of trying for a baby without success.

They told us that my tubes were clear and there were no problems with my husband's sperm count. I had never had troublesome periods – just the occasional slight cramp – and never suspected there might be anything wrong. I was put on the drug Clomid, which stimulates ovulation, for six months and was so desperate to conceive that I asked to continue taking it, even though I was suffering from hot flushes and mood swings.

After about nine months I began to get appalling period pain. I was doubled over and couldn't stand upright so I knew something was wrong. I was fast-tracked for a laparoscopy and they found endometriosis around one of my Fallopian tubes, which was removed using a laser. I couldn't understand how it could have been missed before, and to this day, I wonder if it was triggered by the strong drugs in some way?

We were entitled to three cycles of fertility treatment and I finally conceived via ICSI. Our daughter was born when I was almost 34 and we now accept that she will be our only child. I'm not sure people realize what a toll fertility treatment takes on your life. It's easy to become obsessed.

I have been told that my endometriosis is beginning to grow back but it doesn't give me any problems at the moment. I have been prescribed mefenamic acid to take if I'm in pain but I'm determined not to take it unless I absolutely have to!

## Adoption

For couples who have been unable to conceive either naturally or with the help of fertility treatment, it is important to remember that there is another way of building a family – adoption. The focus of adoption in the twenty-first century is on finding loving homes for children whose birth parents cannot care for them, rather than finding solutions for couples who can't have their own children. Like assisted conception, adoption is not for everyone, but it is right for some couples – and, indeed, some single people – and can prove to be enormously rewarding.

The charity First4Adoption (see Useful addresses) says that there are around 4000 children in the UK looking for new families. They come from a variety of ethnic and religious backgrounds. Over half are sibling groups, some are school age, some have special needs. If you want to adopt you have to be over 21, but there is no upper age limit. You can be married or single, straight or gay, able-bodied or disabled, from any ethnic background, and you don't have to own your own home or be well-off. It is also worth contacting Adoption UK (see Useful addresses) which is a support group for adoptive parents and those planning or hoping to adopt.

# 7

# The age factor

Until fairly recently, endometriosis was thought to affect women in the 20 to 40 age group only. However, research has revealed that it's also possible for teenage girls to have endometriosis. The American Endometriosis Association found that about two-thirds of the women contacting them had experienced problems before they were 20, even though they were rarely actually diagnosed with endometriosis at that age. Likewise, a major international study, published in 2011 by the World Endometriosis Research Foundation (see Useful addresses), involving more than 1400 women in 10 countries, found that one-fifth of them had sought help for their symptoms before they were 19.[2]

At the other end of the age spectrum, it was also thought that the menopause would mean the end of endometriosis symptoms for most women. In theory, that should be the case. Endometriosis is known to be hormone related, so it should produce fewer symptoms after the menopause when women's bodies are producing less oestrogen. Again, that doesn't always happen, and studies carried out in both the USA and Australia have found women still having problems in their later years. Consultant gynaecologist Alfred Cutner, who is the Joint Lead at the Endometriosis Centre at University College Hospital London, says that although there is still much that we don't know about the causes of endometriosis, we do know that it is multifactorial. He says:

> For example, older women in the past had far fewer menstrual cycles over their lifetimes than women do today. They tended to start their periods later and spend much of their adult life either pregnant or breastfeeding – and then died much younger than women do now. Fewer menstrual cycles meant much less endometriosis and the reverse is also true – women today have fewer pregnancies and tend to start their families later so they have more periods over a lifetime.

Endometriosis UK have a booklet called *Is This Normal?*, written to raise awareness among teenagers that they shouldn't suffer crippling period pains without asking for medical help. Of course there are two problems here. Young girls only have experience of their own periods and they can't know what to expect unless they discuss the subject with their mothers, sisters and other girls. Although periods are not a taboo subject any more, many girls are still extremely shy and embarrassed when it comes to anything to do with the way their bodies work and may find it difficult to raise the subject. They may also not want to seem like wimps, or in any way different from their peers. Another difficulty is that, sadly, they may never have heard of Endometriosis UK.

Mums, older sisters, and close friends can do a lot to help. If your daughter, or sister, or friend seems to be having a worse than usual time with her periods every month, you could gently suggest that she ask for help from her GP. Point out that something is not right:

- if she feels ill enough every month to be off school or work, or if she feels faint or nauseous or has to lie down for more than an hour or two;
- if she has – or is afraid she will have – flooding, or accidents because her periods are so heavy, or if she is using tampons plus a sanitary towel and still has to change every couple of hours;
- if she becomes excessively tired, or has pelvic pain all through the month, or pain when she uses the loo.

Sometimes these early-days period pains settle down as her body matures. If they don't, and they continue to cause problems, you might suspect endometriosis. Talk to her about your own periods – if they are within the normal range – and explain that even though it's not unusual to have a bit of pain and discomfort, periods shouldn't be agonizing or stop her from living her usual life. It's normal for girls and women to have some pain for a few hours, maybe even a couple of days, but it's the sort of pain that can be relieved by over-the-counter painkillers, some of which are specially formulated for period pains. Ask your pharmacist's advice.

### How to help with the pain

As well as asking your pharmacist about over-the-counter pain relief, the following suggestions may help.

- Some women find Buscopan helpful, which is more usually recommended for the cramps caused by IBS.
- Make sure the woman isn't constipated and is taking plenty of exercise – a brisk walk or a game of tennis or netball might help even if she doesn't feel much like it.
- It's also important to eat a healthy diet with a special emphasis on essential fatty acids, such as those found in oily fish.
- Vitamin $B_6$, found in wheat germ, wheat bran, cod, turkey, and bananas, and the mineral magnesium, found in nuts and seeds, are also said to help with menstrual cramps. Some women find a magnesium supplement helpful – for maximum effect it should be taken all month round, not just during the period (see page 65).
- It's always a good idea, however old you are, to keep a pain and symptom diary so that when you do go to the doctor, you can give him or her plenty of information. Is the pain a sharp, cramping one, or more of a dull ache? Exactly where in your body is it – your pelvic area, your back and legs, or elsewhere? Does it hurt to use the loo? Do you have other symptoms like fainting or sickness? Do you suffer from mood swings around period time? Do you have unexplained pain between your periods too?
- It's important for young girls to realize that chronic, crippling pelvic pain is not normal or 'just part of being a woman' or 'something you have to put up with each month'. It needs to be taken seriously, and it can be treated. Research in the USA has discovered that if endometriosis in young teenagers is treated early, it tends not to get worse over time, so the sooner young women approach their GP for a diagnosis, the better.

## Help from your doctor

It is common for periods to be trouble-free for the first couple of years and it is only when a young woman begins to ovulate regularly that problems set in. Period pains, often cramp-like, are most usually caused by prostaglandins – chemicals released by the body which make the muscles of the womb contract as they shed the womb lining every month. Consultant gynaecologist Alfred Cutner agrees that not all cases of period pain in teenagers are caused by endometriosis, and that the majority of girls can get help from their GP, with the contraceptive pill as the most usual treatment. He says:

> The combined pill, taken continuously, should help with symptoms because it will mean fewer periods. The pill can be a medical treatment, as well as a contraceptive! Teenagers are only referred to someone like myself if their symptoms don't improve. Endometriosis is a variable condition and usually the impact on young girls is that it affects their school attendance. Usually, the worse the endometriosis, the worse the pain, but that isn't always the case. If the lesions are in an area where there are a lot of nerve fibres, then the pain will tend to be worse. I ask them lots of questions so that I get a full picture of the pain they are in and where and when it occurs. I may also have to ask if they are sexually active and, if they are, whether they have deep pain during sex. I may then have to give them an internal examination and/or a vaginal scan which will reveal any nodules or cysts, with surgery as a last resort.

Eighteen-year-old Alice shared her story on ITV's *This Morning* during 2014's Endometriosis Awareness Week. She said:

> I began having severe pain when I was 12 before my periods had even started. When they did, the pain became worse. My periods were heavy and painful and on one occasion the school bus had to be diverted to Accident and Emergency because I was so ill. I was put on a morphine drip. This kept happening until I was in pain for most of the month. I became anaemic and was terribly tired all the time, but it was still two and a half years before endometriosis was diagnosed. I hadn't heard of it and although I was relieved when I finally learned what was wrong, I was upset when I learned that it might lead to infertility. I felt I had been robbed of my rights as a woman.

Amy started her periods at 13 and was prescribed anti-depressants and told her symptoms were psychological!

> I always struggled and couldn't understand how it was that my friends seemed to sail through that time of the month when I felt so awful every time. I was sure something was wrong when I was rolling around on the floor with pain, crying, being sick and having to take time off school.

It was only when I went back to my GP after I'd had random bleeding when I went to the loo that I was referred to a gynaecologist. I was put on the pill at first, which did help, but then the random bleeding began again and I had a laparoscopy when I was 19 which revealed Stage II endometriosis.

## Menopause and after

As we have already seen, in theory, endometriosis symptoms should become less troublesome after the menopause, whatever kind of treatment you have had, or even if you have managed without treatment at all. Endometriosis causes fewer problems for most women after the menopause because their bodies are producing very little oestrogen. However, there's now evidence that not every woman's symptoms disappear after the menopause. For an unlucky few women there may still be pelvic pain, however, because the endometriosis has caused adhesions and scarring to their pelvic organs. The ovaries may be stuck down, the bowel may be twisted or the ureter (the tube which carries urine between the kidneys and the bladder) may be compressed and this can cause pain. Or, it is always possible that there may be inflammation in the area from other causes.

Some research studies have found that endometriosis can cause problems even in post-menopausal women, and may return if you are prescribed HRT. So how does this happen? Fluctuating hormone levels during the menopause or the peri-menopause – the years before your periods actually stop – can cause irregular bleeding or an unpredictably heavy flow. Even after the menopause, if you still have your ovaries, they will be producing a small amount of oestrogen and this could be enough to cause problems in susceptible women. A total hysterectomy, of course, where the ovaries are removed as well as the womb and other organs, should prevent this happening, unless any ovarian tissue is mistakenly left in the pelvic area.

# HRT

It seems logical to assume that HRT, often prescribed for women who have unbearable menopausal symptoms such as hot flushes, night sweats, vaginal dryness and mood swings, could have an effect on endometriosis symptoms, even though the dose of oestrogen prescribed is relatively small. HRT is still something of a controversial treatment for menopausal and post-menopausal women anyway, with women usually being told that they need to weigh up the benefits (fewer menopausal symptoms, some protection against coronary heart disease and osteoporosis) against the disadvantages (a slightly increased risk of breast cancer). If you add endometriosis to the mix, it seems as though the decision will be even more difficult for individual women and their doctors.

If a woman is prescribed HRT, her doctor should be made aware that she has – or has had – endometriosis. Michael Dooley, consultant gynaecologist at the Poundbury Clinics, says:

A lot will depend on the type of HRT which is prescribed. A sequential type – where the woman takes oestrogen every day and progestogen for 12 to 14 days at the end of her menstrual cycle – might have a negative effect, but a course of continuous combined HRT – where she takes oestrogen and progestogen every day – should be okay, though this is a poorly researched area. As with many forms of treatment, the benefits have to be weighed up against the risks. Management of the condition very much depends on the individual woman. For example, if endometriosis has left adhesions on her bowel then a healthy diet which helps her to avoid bloating and constipation can be helpful. The only other option would be surgery.

Some researchers have suggested that the fact that some older women still have endometriosis could indicate that it's not about oestrogen production at all – or only partly. Given that relatively little is known about the causes of endometriosis, they could have a point (see Chapter 3). Perhaps the possibility that the immune system is involved, or environmental toxins, or each woman's lifestyle, diet and habits, could have something to do with it?

Treatment of post-menopausal women with endometriosis clearly needs to take into account the possible side effects of hormonal drugs on women in this age group. There doesn't seem to be any consensus about what type of HRT is most suitable for women with endometriosis after their menopause, whether they have a natural menopause or a surgical one after a hysterectomy. If any patches of endometriosis remain in the pelvic cavity after the operation, then taking oestrogen-only HRT may mean that the condition returns. Taking combined HRT (oestrogen/progestogen), however, may slightly increase your risk of developing breast cancer. The increased risk is small in women under normal menopause age – around 51 – but slightly higher for older women. So any decision to take HRT must be a matter for each individual and her doctors to decide.

Alfred Cutner points out that, whereas it is perfectly acceptable for a 17-year-old to be prescribed the pill on a continuous basis so that she has fewer periods, this wouldn't be advised for someone aged 50 because of the known side effects of hormone treatments on post-menopausal women. He says:

> If a patient needed HRT because of her menopausal symptoms and she had had a radical hysterectomy because of endometriosis, I would be inclined to prescribe nothing for four or five months to give her body a chance to settle down after the operation. After that I might prescribe Livial – which is a combined oestrogen/progestogen HRT tablet – for six months to a year, and oestrogen-only HRT after that. But it does depend very much on the individual, there are no real hard and fast rules.

## Connie

Connie is now in her sixties and says she no longer has any pelvic pain at all and is fitter and healthier than she has ever been. She was only diagnosed with endometriosis after being treated for breast cancer when she was 37, and wonders if the hormonal treatments she had for the cancer somehow triggered the development of endometriosis.

> I did have very painful periods when I was a teenager. They lasted about six days and I had to take time off school. My doctor suggested a cocktail of painkillers which did help, as did hugging a hot-water bottle. No-one ever suggested endometriosis. Perhaps in those days no-one thought of it? I was on the pill for a time and then married and had my

children. I had no special problems getting pregnant though I did have several miscarriages. When I was expecting my daughter I had a lot of bleeding and had to have progesterone injections and take it very easy.

Then, when I was 37, I found a lump and cancer was diagnosed. I was told I would have to take tamoxifen for five years to prevent any recurrence. That was when the severe pain started. I had periods which lasted ten days and were extremely painful. I can remember having to stop driving my car and lie down in the back seat because I was in so much pain! I had to stay in bed and was fit for nothing.

I had a laparoscopy which revealed endometriosis. Various treatments were tried including Danazol but that produced such bad side effects I was advised to stop taking it. I then had laser treatment in Birmingham Women's Hospital and that seemed to do the trick. I was probably approaching the menopause at that time anyway and I could tolerate the remaining periods. My menopause itself wasn't stressful, I didn't have any symptoms like hot flushes or anxiety or depression and was so relieved not to be in pain any longer!

Whatever your age, management of endometriosis must be tailored to your own individual circumstances, including factors such as whether you are hoping to have children in the future or have completed your family. Consultant gynaecologist Michael Dooley says:

A woman with endometriosis, whatever her age, might need support and counselling because of the effects on her daily life, her sex life and her fertility, and this support might involve gastroenterologists, urologists, and psychologists as well as gynaecologists. There may also be a place for complementary therapies too.

We shall be looking at self-help and complementary therapies in the next chapters. There is still a lot we don't know about endometriosis, but we can offer help in managing the condition and trying to prevent it getting worse.

# 8

# Lifestyle changes

Lifestyle factors are an important part of treating endometriosis. You owe it to yourself to be as fit and healthy as possible. No-one feels their best if they are poorly nourished, inactive, and suffering from stress and lack of refreshing sleep. Taking care of your health puts you in control, not the endometriosis, and that can have a positive psychological effect. Because the effects of endometriosis on women's lives vary so much, an integrated approach often works really well. In addition to help and support from the medical profession, self-help can be a powerful tool to help manage endometriosis and your general health and well-being.

## An endometriosis-friendly diet?

Research indicates that some women are helped by reducing the amount of red meat, wheat and dairy in their diets. Several studies from the USA and Europe recommend diets rich in vegetables, nuts and seeds. One US study found that women who drank more than two cups of coffee a day were twice as likely to have endometriosis as those who drank two cups or fewer.[4] Italian researchers found that women who ate red meat every day were at twice the risk of endometriosis of women who only ate red meat three times a week, and that women who ate more than 14 portions of fruit and vegetables a week are 70 per cent less likely to have endometriosis than those who ate fewer than six portions.[5] So, drinking less coffee and eating more vegetables and fruit seem like wise choices. Consultant gynaecologist Michael Dooley, of the Poundbury Clinics, recommends that those who come to see him follow a diet containing foods rich in folic acid – that means greens like broccoli, spinach, kale and dark-leaved cabbage and lettuce.

### Endometriosis and trans-fats

Women whose diets are high in trans-fatty acids have nearly a 50 per cent higher chance of developing endometriosis than those whose diets are low in these fats, according to findings from the US Nurses Health Study. Researchers at the Brigham and Women's Hospital and Harvard Medical School in Boston MA followed almost 71,000 US nurses for 12 years. The researchers were looking at the effects of fat consumption on endometriosis and found that the women's total fat intake did not seem to be linked to endometriosis. However, when they looked at the type of fat eaten, there did seem to be a link.

- Women with a high intake of omega-3 fatty acids – the kind of fat which is found in oily fish such as salmon, herring, mackerel and sardines – were much less likely to develop endometriosis.
- The top fifth of oily fish consumers (those who ate most oily fish) were 22 per cent less likely to have endometriosis than the bottom fifth (those who ate least oily fish).
- The US researchers found that the top fifth of trans-fat consumers (the women who ate the most trans-fats) were 48 per cent more likely to have endometriosis than the bottom fifth (those who ate least trans-fats).

Trans-fats are fats treated by a process known as hydrogenation, to give them a longer shelf-life. Fast foods and commercially produced pies and cakes are likely to list hydrogenated fats or trans-fats among their ingredients – just look at the labels.

## Avoiding constipation

If you have bowel adhesions, which make going to the loo very painful, then it's extremely important that you don't allow yourself to become constipated.

- A healthy diet with plenty of fruit and vegetables and plain water to prevent dehydration will keep you regular without having to resort to laxatives.
- Include more fibre in your diet – but build your intake up slowly as eating too much at once may cause bloating and wind.
- Take regular gentle exercise.

- Take your time. Feelings of being stressed and harried can militate against regular bowel habits.
- Everyone has their favourite anti-constipation foods, but some suggestions include: a small bowl of All-Bran, two or three dried figs or dates, a handful of cherries, some prunes, or beans on toast.

## Supplements

Vitamins and minerals can, of course, be obtained from the food we eat, but some women like to give their diets a boost by taking vitamin supplements. In either case, if you have endometriosis you might the following helpful.

- Vitamin $B_6$, found in wheat germ, wheat bran, bananas and green veg, can help with PMS-type symptoms, depression and fatigue.
- Vitamin $B_{12}$, found in bran, eggs and cereals, can help improve mood and is especially important for vegetarians as a strict vegetarian diet contains little of this vitamin.
- Magnesium, found in seeds, nuts and bran, can help ease period cramps especially when taken alongside Vitamin $B_6$.
- Zinc, found in oysters, wheat germ and pumpkin seeds can help boost immunity.

### Get tested for anaemia

If, despite eating a good diet, you find yourself getting easily tired and breathless, have a pale complexion, and frequently feel faint, it may be worth getting yourself tested for anaemia caused by heavy periods. This is a simple, commonly performed blood test to measure the amount of haemoglobin in your blood. Many doctors believe that anaemia is best treated as a symptom rather than a condition in its own right – that is, the underlying cause of the anaemia should always be found and treated. However, meanwhile you can boost your iron intake by consuming foods rich in iron, such as bran, dried apricots and tuna as well as red meat. A gentle supplement such as Floradix or Spatone may help. Iron can help ease period pains as well as improving anaemia.

- Calcium, found in dairy products, sesame seeds and sardines, can help with cramps and pelvic pain.
- Selenium, found in Brazil nuts, fish and wholemeal bread, can stimulate the immune system.
- Co-enzyme $Q_{10}$, found in seafood and wholegrains, can have an anti-ageing effect.

## A nutritional approach to endometriosis

Maryon Stewart is a pioneer in non-drug medicine who set up the Women's Nutritional Advisory Service – later called the Natural Health Advisory Service – in 1984 (see Useful addresses). Over the years she has successfully treated thousands of women with hormone-based health problems, from PMS to the menopause, offering advice on diet changes.

Hormone-related problems, ranging from PMS to the menopause, are treated with a diet containing regular, small amounts of naturally occurring plant oestrogens, also known as phyto-oestrogens. These compounds are plant nutrients which exert an oestrogen-like effect on the body, although they are, Maryon points out, one thousand times less potent. They have a balancing effect on the body's hormone levels, raising the levels if they are too low, but lowering them if oestrogen dominance is a problem, as it may be in women with endometriosis. Phyto-oestrogens are found in soya and soya products; for example, flour, tofu, soya milk, golden linseeds and the herb, red clover. Maryon's diet programme recommends consuming these little and often throughout the day.

She recommends a diet which is high in fibre and low in animal fat to prevent oestrogen surges. It helps if you eat plenty of nuts and seeds – linseeds, sunflower seeds, flax and pumpkin seeds – as they also contain essential fatty acids, which help to relieve pain and inflammation. Bread with added soya and linseeds is widely available and you can sprinkle seeds on breakfast cereals and salads. Maryon also recommends:

- supplements – a multi-vitamin and mineral, 300 mg of magnesium per day, plus evening primrose oil and marine fish oil which helps to regulate hormones and also has anti-inflammatory properties. Zinc supplements are necessary for the correct metabolism of essential fatty acids, and consumption of wheat products should be reduced as they can inhibit absorption of zinc.

- plenty of vegetables – organic if possible.
- a reduction in the amount of meat and high-fat dairy products you consume.
- a gradual change in diet, rather than suddenly swapping a traditional meat and two veg, high-fat, sugar-rich diet for something healthier! Take it slowly and give your body time to adjust.

## Keep moving!

Physical activity improves your general well-being and can have a positive impact on your symptoms.

- Exercise produces endorphins, the feel-good hormones which help to raise your spirits.
- Around ten minutes of moderate exercise (that makes you breathe hard) is all you need to start producing endorphins.
- Exercise lowers the amount of oestrogen in the body, which may help improve symptoms (lowering oestrogen is the aim of much endometriosis treatment).
- Exercise helps to keep a sluggish digestive system moving which again can help to improve symptoms.
- Exercise improves circulation, gets the heart pumping and improves the blood flow to our organs.

### Becoming more active

Perhaps the simplest way to begin is by incorporating more exercise into your everyday life. That way you are likely to achieve the recommended 30 minutes a day almost without noticing! It's easier if you travel to work by public transport. Just get on the bus a stop or two further away from home or walk to a slightly more distant train or Underground station. Don't take the lift or escalator; walk up the stairs instead. If you travel by car, make a point of parking at the far end of the car park. More and more people are choosing to walk or cycle or jog to work these days. Or, take yourself out of the office at lunch time and walk through the nearest park or along the river or canal bank. You could start a lunchtime challenge in your office to see how far you and your colleagues could get in the

### How much exercise?

Some studies suggest that exercise has to be done at a certain pitch if it is to be beneficial – that is, that it needs to be done at a certain intensity and for a certain amount of time if it is to have any protective effect against endometriosis. Doing at least four hours exercise a week would appear to be the tipping point to feel the benefits, according to a study by Dr Lisa Signorello and colleagues of the Brigham Women's Hospital, Boston. The study suggested that exercise needs to be frequent, regular and vigorous to be effective.

Other research has also indicated that exercise needs to be of a reasonable intensity. One study, by researchers Dr Preet Dhillon and Dr Victoria Holt, who is professor in epidemiology at the University of Washington, states that women who participate in regular, high-intensity physical activity such as running, biking, swimming and playing tennis have a 75 per cent reduction in the risk of developing endometriosis as compared to women who did not participate in any form of exercise. Irregular exercise, or low-intensity exercise did not appear to have the same benefits in this study.[6] However, you should by no means wait for the perfect exercise programme to materialize – any form of exercise is beneficial. Endometriosis and fertility expert Michael Dooley recommends that you undertake any form of exercise that you enjoy. The message is to keep as mobile as possible and to build physical activity into your life. Anything you can manage is better than nothing, and can always be built up in small increments. 'Anything which improves your general well-being, makes you happy and helps you to cope with the chronic pain, is worth doing,' says Mr Dooley.

allowed time. In your free time, explore your town or city, with your partner and family if you like. Gardening and housework can count as exercise. Do a bit of bending and stretching while you're waiting for the kettle to boil or the microwave to ping. It all helps to keep you moving.

### Which exercise?

There are literally hundreds of different kinds of exercise you can try, whether it is dancing, swimming, skating, playing tennis or golf – or simply walking! Ask yourself some questions – would you prefer to exercise indoors or is being out in the fresh air more your thing? Do you fancy the idea of team sports, joining a walking group or keep fit class with others, or going for a run or swim on your own? A quick look at your local Council's website will give you an idea of the exercise opportunities in your area, many of which are free or very low-cost. Many gyms and swimming pools run women-only sessions, mum-and-baby, or older people sessions, which suit anyone who might feel self-conscious about not having exercised for some time. Have you considered:

- jogging, keep fit, aerobics, step classes, trampolining, fencing, basketball, tennis, swimming, aqua-aerobics, women's football or rugby, ballroom dancing, line dancing, salsa, country-dancing or folk-dancing, golf, cycling, rambling, spinning, Pilates, power-walking, dry skiing, Nordic walking, Boxercise, ballet, Fitball, rowing, netball, disco or jazz dance, ice-skating, kick-boxing, martial arts, rollerblading, snowboarding, hockey, Body Conditioning, skipping, squash, hiking, pole-dancing, British Military Fitness, Slimnastics, lacrosse, table-tennis, badminton, climbing, scuba-diving, riding, walking a dog (your own or someone else's)?

There must be something in that list which appeals? Or, you could just buy a fitness DVD which enables you to work out in your own front room. Choose an exercise regime you actually enjoy! This is vital. So many people join gyms in January as part of a New Year resolution, then lose interest and stop attending. Not only is that an expensive mistake but it's also demoralizing. Exercise has to be something you like and look forward to, or you won't keep it up. If you think you hate it, or have *never* found anything that didn't seem like a chore, think again!

## Connie

Connie, who is in her sixties, was advised by a female doctor to take up an exercise regime when she was experiencing severe pain linked to endometriosis and says she feels fitter than she has ever been.

> I was unable to work full-time because the pain was unpredictable, though I did do some part-time supply teaching. My doctor said that

joining a gym would be the best thing I could do as exercise would let the endorphins kick in. There was so much choice. I ended up doing water aerobics, Pilates, yoga and line dancing and it turned out to be the best thing I could have done. Exercise definitely lifts your spirits even when you are in pain!

### Can exercise be dangerous?

One or two researchers have expressed concern that vigorous exercise during menstruation might encourage the development of endometriosis by increasing the chances of retrograde menstruation, but there is very little evidence to support this. On the contrary, most research suggests that exercise decreases the risk of endometriosis by reducing levels of oestrogen and possible endometrial aromatase activity.[7]

It's more likely that some women simply feel too uncomfortable and shattered to exercise during their period. In which case, it's important not to feel guilty. Just resume your normal levels of physical activity when you feel able. The only other slight risk involved is if you become so hooked on exercise that you over-do it and run the risk of injury. If you feel this does pose a danger, discuss it with a physiotherapist, an adviser at your local gym, your doctor, or a therapist.

## Relaxation

In today's fast-paced world where we tend to do everything at a run, and carry our smartphones everywhere, even on holiday, the idea of relaxation can sometimes seem like an impossible dream. But if you are battling a chronic illness, learning to relax is even more essential than it is for people who don't have a health problem. Pain makes your body tense up, and the more tense you are, the worse the pain can be.

### So what are the best ways to relax?

As with exercise, you can start simple. Accept that you have a right to 'me time', however busy your life may be. Running yourself into the ground to benefit your employer or your family is counter-productive because it will result in burn-out. Half an hour with a magazine and a cup of tea, a warm bath scented with your favourite essential oil, five minutes deep, regular breathing with your eyes closed, taking you away to a favourite place in your mind, can all be remarkably therapeutic. Other ways to relax are discussed below.

## Yoga

Yoga, which may have been practised as a therapy for as long as five thousand years, is well-known to aid relaxation and reduce stress. The word yoga is derived from a Sanskrit word meaning union. The idea is to promote well-being by bringing mind, body – including the hormonal system – and spirit into a perfectly balanced state by means of exercise, correct breathing and meditation. Like other relaxation therapies, yoga does help in managing endometriosis.

Yoga has been popular in the UK since Victorian times, with a resurgence of interest in the hippie 60s. Classes in the various kinds of yoga are widely available all over the country and you can find out more about what is on offer from the British Wheel of Yoga (see Useful addresses). It is possible to practise yoga on your own or accompanied by a DVD, but it's often more beneficial to join a class and be guided by an experienced teacher.

The British Wheel website points out that yoga is something everyone can practise, whatever their age, gender or state of health, and that it can provide tools which enable you to cope with the challenges of daily life. It promotes relaxation, increases your sense of well-being, and can help combat anxiety and depression. Yoga classes are non-competitive which means everyone works at their own level. Particular postures or asanas are recommended for women with gynaecological problems, including endometriosis. Ask the class teacher about the Upside Down Seal or the Bridge posture.

## Autogenic training

Autogenic training (AT) is another relaxation therapy which is less widely known than yoga but which can be very successful in combatting the stress which is caused by chronic illness and pain. AT consists of a simple series of mental exercises devised by a German doctor about a hundred years ago. These exercises are designed to switch off the stress-producing fight-or-flight response, which can affect every part of your body, and to replace it with the gentle rest-and-relax response instead. The key point about AT is that you don't have to try to do anything, not even let your mind go blank or chase away intrusive thoughts. You simply, as one of the exercises puts it, 'become your own passive observer'. Counselling psychologist Stephen Ashby says, 'The course helps individuals to create a calm centre, and once you learn the basics, it's with you forever. It's there, within yourself, that's what the word "autogenic" means.'

AT is normally taught in a series of eight weekly classes. Once you have learned the exercises you can practise them at any time that you feel yourself becoming stressed. By releasing unnecessary tension in all parts of your body, it can help with pain relief, stress and insomnia. You can learn more about it from the website <www.autogenic-therapy.org.uk> (see Useful addresses).

## Mindfulness

Mindfulness is a technique which involves accepting life as it is and living in the moment. Through meditation you learn to find a place of stillness within yourself, to focus on the present and take time to look at what is happening around you in a totally non-judgemental way. You become aware of your thoughts, feelings and sensations and learn to accept them. A study at Oxford University found that mindfulness courses were not only helpful in reducing anxiety and stress, but also could have a positive effect on physical conditions such as chronic pain and even high blood pressure. A pilot study, Mindfulness-based psychological intervention for coping with pain in endometriosis, by Mette Kold and colleagues of Aalborg University, Denmark, has suggested that mindfulness techniques are helpful for coping with endometriosis.[8] Although more research is needed, preliminary results indicate significant and lasting effects on pain levels, well-being, and ability to function in daily life. The findings are in line with qualitative studies in women with endometriosis, and with data on the effects of mindfulness in other chronic pain domains. Mindfulness is well-documented to have a beneficial effect on chronic pain conditions. A review of 133 studies between 1960 to 2010 carried out by Keren Reiner and colleagues of Ben Gurion University of the Negev, Israel, selected 16 studies that indicated that mindful practices may indeed reduce pain intensity in those with chronic pain conditions.[9]

## The importance of sleep

In addition to a healthy diet, exercise, and relaxation, another component of well-being is deep, refreshing sleep. Like true relaxation, this is difficult to achieve if you are in constant pain. Ironically, the more you worry about not being able to sleep, the less likely you are to sleep soundly. The relaxation therapies mentioned above all help to promote sound sleep, with autogenic training being especially successful. Here are some tips to help you to sleep better.

- Remember that people all need different amounts of sleep. If you wake up most mornings feeling refreshed and ready for the day, you are probably getting enough, even if this is not the recommended 7–8 hours.
- Make sure your bedroom is sleep-friendly – it's amazing how many are not! You don't need a TV, mobile phone or any other electronic device in your bedroom. It's for sleep (and sex) and that's all! It should be dark, warm (but not too hot) and quiet. How long is it since you bought a new bed? One that is too hard, too soft, or just uncomfortable should be replaced if possible. The same goes for pillows.
- Avoid heavy meals for four or five hours before you go to bed. A disturbed digestion is almost guaranteed to stop you sleeping. The traditional warm, milky drink can help – milk contains the amino acid tryptophan which is a sleep aid. Avoid caffeine too.
- Realize that an alcoholic nightcap is not a good idea. You might fall asleep more easily but you are likely to wake in the small hours with a full bladder and be unable to go to sleep again.
- Only go to bed when you feel tired, and consider reading (no thrillers!) or simply relaxing from your toes to the top of your head before you drop off.
- Get up and do something boring if you are wide awake in the middle of the night, rather than tossing and turning and fretting because you are not asleep yet.
- Sleeping pills can be helpful in the short-term but it's better not to rely on them. By all means ask your GP for help with insomnia though. Chronic insomniacs can often be referred to sleep clinics for specialist help.

# 9

# Complementary medicine

If you are living with any chronic condition, especially one for which conventional medicine is limited, it can be tempting to go for an alternative or complementary approach. If you have suffered for years and nothing your GP has suggested has proved helpful, what do you have to lose? In addition, many women are reluctant to take powerful drugs which are proven to have side effects, and the thought of surgery can be frightening. Consulting a complementary practitioner such as a homoeopath or acupuncturist can seem like an appealing alternative.

Most complementary therapists work holistically – that is, they look at the person they are treating as a whole, investigating their medical history, personality, mental and emotional issues as well as painful periods or fertility problems. Within the medical profession, opinions on complementary therapy are still divided, and some doctors dismiss alternative treatments as so much superstition or mumbo-jumbo. They point out that pharmaceutical drugs have to go through rigorous, double-blind, placebo-controlled trials before they are even put on the market. Complementary remedies often don't – and when they are subjected to the same rigorous testing process, they fail. Any success is put down to the placebo effect as it is known that, in some cases, people will say they feel better if they are given *any* treatment, even if this involves harmless pills with no active ingredient at all! The NHS Choices website says that the placebo effect is 'a phenomenon that we don't completely understand. But we can see it working in all kinds of ways'.

Others in the medical profession are more open-minded, realizing that people are more than just collections of symptoms, and that a more holistic approach to treatment can be beneficial. They acknowledge that some complementary medicines appear to help some people with some conditions, and especially those for whom scientific medicine has not yet found the answers. They also recognize that some complementary remedies and treatments, for instance homoeopathy and reflexology, are always prescribed on an individual basis. This means that two women with endometriosis who consult a qualified homoeopath or reflexologist will not necessarily be given the same remedy or the same treatment. This makes the sort of clinical trials described above very difficult to carry out. Medical herbalists, too, base their treatment choices on many years of practical experience. Recognized complementary treatments that help with pain management, or aid relaxation, are likely to be beneficial. From the sufferer's point of view, it doesn't matter a bit whether this is the result of the placebo effect or something else. You just want to feel better!

If you do go down the alternative route, however, it's important that you consult a reputable practitioner. There are regulatory bodies for homoeopaths, herbalists, acupuncturists and other complementary therapists and, before you consult anyone, you should make sure that they are appropriately qualified.

## Acupuncture

Acupuncture, which has been practised in China and other Eastern countries for millennia, is generally thought of as a system of pain relief, and can be used to treat a variety of different illnesses and conditions. It is a holistic therapy, whose aim is to restore the whole body to its natural balance and good health.

Traditional Chinese medicine is based on completely different principles from the medicine we know in the West. The Chinese believe that health depends on *Qi* – the body's own energy or life force – flowing smoothly in channels beneath the skin, known as meridians. Illness results from blockages and lack of balance in these channels. Acupuncture is said to restore the balance by inserting very fine needles into these channels to stimulate a healing response. There have been some scientific studies, mostly in China, which support acupuncture as a treatment for endometriosis. It can provide pain relief, stimulating the nerves and leading to the release of endorphins. It also seems to reduce inflammation and regulates the levels of prostaglandins.

A consultation with an acupuncturist will consist of a detailed conversation with you, asking about your general health – both physical, mental and emotional – as well as about the problem that has brought you along. You will also be asked about your medical history and that of your family, your pulse will be taken and your tongue examined. This all enables the therapist to work out the best treatment for you as an individual, before very fine needles are inserted into the appropriate acupuncture point – which may not be anywhere near the site of your pain! Acupuncture should not be painful. If you are needle-phobic, similar effects can be obtained by burning a herb called moxa to warm up the acupuncture points, and massage can also be used.

Traditional Chinese medicine (TCM) would be likely to diagnose blood stasis as a cause of endometriosis – in other words, an imbalance in the flow of *Qi* or natural energy. As well as acupuncture, Chinese herbs would probably be prescribed and, interestingly, a low-fat, dairy-free diet. In 2009, Southampton University researchers looked at the studies which had been done in China itself, where TCM is a routine treatment for women with endometriosis and is said to offer both pain relief and an improvement in fertility. The British researchers thought that TCM seemed to be as effective as some of the strong drugs prescribed in this country and produced fewer side effects. However, they only looked at a relatively small number of research studies involving 158 women, and said that more research was needed. They also pointed out that it is very important that anyone consulting a Chinese physician in this country makes sure that they are properly qualified, ideally in Western medicine as well as TCM. The Acumedic Chinese medical centre in North London has been established for more than 40 years and is a good place to start (see Useful addresses).

Judy Elliott (see Useful addresses) is an acupuncturist, who trained at the College of Integrated Chinese Medicine in Reading, and likes to work alongside traditionally trained Western doctors as well as herbalists, osteopaths and other complementary therapists. She used acupuncture herself to help with her back problems. Judy finds that some 70 per cent of her clients are women, many of whom consult her about gynaecological problems, including endometriosis, when they have not found more conventional approaches to treatment helpful. She says:

Hormonal issues are not well catered for in any medical system, and we don't yet know exactly what causes endometriosis although there are a number of theories. Complementary therapists use detailed consultations with their patients to build up a picture of what is happening. There are a number of factors involved – most illnesses have more than a single cause! There is usually an underlying hormonal imbalance which may be partly hereditary. Oestrogen dominance plays a part. There may be environmental links – I treated a woman who grew up next to a fertilizer plant where the fields were constantly being sprayed. There may have been physical trauma – operations can lead to adhesions – or psychological trauma.

In Chinese medicine, 'Five Elements Acupuncture' will look at emotions as well as physical symptoms. Anger, worry and stress can eat away at your constitution. Negative emotions like frustration and resentment are driven by the liver. There are eight syndromes for endometriosis in Chinese medicine. 'Blood stagnation' means that the blood does not flow properly which is why, in a consultation, I will ask for a lot of detail about the woman's periods – is the blood thin and light in colour, or thick and sticky? Are there a lot of clots? Is her cycle short or long? Where exactly is the pain and what type of pain is it? I look at the woman's constitution, whether she is hot or cold, when and what she eats, how well her digestion works. This all brings an added dimension to the diagnosis.

Acupuncture tends to be a long-term treatment and yes, it works – women experience remission of their pain which is what they want. I need to see three cycles before I can make a diagnosis. Acupuncture is used to support the woman's menstrual cycle with different treatments at different times of the month to support the healthy flow of blood, possibly using Chinese herbs as well if there is a lot of blood stagnation. I work out a treatment regime with my patients and see where we go!

Rosemary is one of Judith's patients. She says that when they met, she felt she had run out of options for treating her endometriosis. She says:

I had had problems since I was in my twenties, with very heavy periods, clotting, severe cramps and hormone-related migraines. After a laparoscopy, laser treatment and six months of hormone injections which left me feeling dreadful, I was ready to try anything. I'd had some acupuncture before, for a different condition, so I thought I would give it a go.

Each time I saw Judith I was asked about everything that was going on in my life – all my symptoms, where I was in my menstrual cycle, my feelings, including the fact I felt it was ruining my life! The sessions were very intense and the treatment regulated my periods so they became lighter and less painful, with no clots. My migraines also cleared up. I still have a treatment every month or so and I find that if I don't the migraines come back.

## Herbal medicine

At one time, all medicine was herbal, and many parts of the world today rely on herbal remedies. Traditional herbalists have learned from many years of experience that herbs can be used to treat all kinds of ailments. Many familiar drugs are based on plant ingredients – aspirin derives from willow bark, morphine from the opium poppy – and some of the modern drugs used to treat cancer and Alzheimer's disease also have plant origins. Buscopan, mentioned in the previous chapter as a possible treatment for abdominal cramps, is derived from the leaves of an Australian shrub.

Herbal remedies can be bought over the counter from health food stores but for a detailed consultation it's worth getting in touch with a qualified medical herbalist through the National Institute of Medical Herbalists <www.nimh.org.uk>. Please also check with your doctor if you are going to take any herbal remedies, especially if you are on regular medications – some medications interact with herbal remedies – or if you have other health conditions. Medical herbalist Hananja Brice-Ytsma from North London says:

> Herbs are just part of the solution. Women have to do some of the work themselves! I always look at diet and exercise as well as prescribing. If you can afford it, I would recommend organic produce and a diet with plenty of vegetables. Fish oils – providing the fish is hormone-free – also have an anti-inflammatory effect. If a woman has been very sedentary I recommend exercise as the pelvic area really needs good circulation. Belly-dancing or exercising with a hula-hoop can help!

Different herbal treatments will be prescribed for every woman, after a detailed consultation. I do have some favourites which I use to support the liver, the immune system, and a healthy circulation, as well as uterine stimulants. Dandelion can work well for oestrogen dominance and liver clearance and it works as a gentle laxative too. Marigold can be prescribed to aid the lymphatic system. Black cohosh is a good anti-inflammatory and black haw works well for uterine cramping, or I might prescribe anemone or pulsatilla for pain.

I am trying to correct the underlying situation so once the symptoms are under control I will try and wean a patient off the herbs. It could take as little as six months to see an improvement or as much as one to two years.

## Homoeopathy

Homoeopathy is a 200-year-old form of complementary medicine which is designed to stimulate the body's own healing processes. Like most complementary treatments, it is based on a holistic, whole-body approach so every treatment plan is tailored to the individual and takes into account someone's personality, background, previous medical history and mental and emotional health as well as their physical symptoms. It is based on the principle that 'like cures like' – something which, in large doses, creates the symptoms will, in small doses, cure it. Homoeopathic medicines are also extremely diluted to eliminate side effects.

Mollie Hunton is a retired GP who developed an interest in homoeopathy because, in her own words, 'I was tired of treating patients who were not getting better!' She is President of the Midlands branch of the Faculty of Homoeopathy and has taught the subject to medical students at Birmingham Medical School. She says:

Women with endometriosis come to me because their conventional treatment isn't working or is causing them troublesome side effects. I started quite tentatively and had some notable successes, including one lady who had been told she had no chance of getting pregnant because of her ovarian cysts. I treated her homoeopathically and she conceived naturally. I need to know all about my patients – their past history, life events, even including what they do for a living, because what you do for a living relates to what is going on in your body. If you are dealing with a bullying boss, for example, the stress of that will lead to suppressed anger, which affects your whole system, and I will treat for that.

What homoeopathy has taught me is to look at patients as individuals and ask why they have their endometriosis – and why now? I've treated women from teenagers to those in their forties. Because they are all different, I may prescribe a different remedy for each woman, depending on her individual needs. I also recommend a sugar-free and dairy-free diet and soya products which provide plant oestrogens. When I looked at those patients who had had a recurrence of symptoms later, I found that they had either had some sort of stressful event in their lives or had dietary lapses.

## Reflexology

Reflexology is a complementary therapy which is based on the idea that certain points on the feet, lower legs, hands, face or ears correspond to different areas of the body. Gentle pressure applied to the appropriate points may restore the body's natural balance, help it to heal itself and reduce stress, promoting better health and helping the person to relax and sleep more soundly. For some women, this gentle therapy can improve symptoms. London reflexologist Tracey Smith (see Useful addresses) says:

It isn't known exactly how reflexology works, although some recent scientific research from Japan, using a functional MRI scanner, has shown a strong correlation between pressure on the peripherals – feet, hands, face or ears – and a change in blood flow to the brain. Women come to me either because they have experienced the benefits of reflexology for another condition, or because they have tried everything else. I am happy to work alongside conventional medicine. Like other complementary therapies, reflexology helps the body to heal itself. People are more than just collections of symptoms and everything in the body is interlinked. I take a full medical history and ask a lot of lifestyle questions about things like diet, exercise and sleep. An initial treatment lasts an hour and is similar, whatever the patient's symptoms are. I can feel which parts of their body are out of balance and what I feel in their feet may not necessarily be the problem they first told me about. The relationship between patient and therapist is very important and I would say that if you don't get on with the person treating you, you should find someone else. My clients make the decision about how often they see me – perhaps weekly at first, then monthly, then when the seasons change. Your body will tell you what you need.

Ruby, whose story was told in Chapter 1 of this book, found that reflexology, plus some dietary changes prescribed by a herbalist, was much more successful in treating her endometriosis than any of the conventional treatments she was offered. She says:

I was recommended to Tracey by a friend. I had had reflexology before with a therapist who didn't speak to me and this was a totally different experience. I noticed an energy boost straight away and the first period I had after the reflexology was completely different. It lasted four days instead of almost a week and was much less painful. I had weekly treatments – seven altogether – and month by month I could see an improvement.

## Osteopathy

The principle behind this therapy is that the body's well-being depends on the skeleton, muscles, ligaments and connective tissues working smoothly together. An osteopath will use touch, manipulation, stretch and massage to restore your body to a state of balance and help it to heal itself, and will also offer some guidance on diet and exercise. It is a safe, natural approach to healthcare, with treatment tailored to the individual, and you can find out more about it from the General Osteopathic Council (see Useful addresses). Most of us probably associate osteopathy with treatment for bad backs and it may be surprising to hear that it can also be used to treat gynaecological conditions like endometriosis. However, osteopaths believe that structure and function are related, in any part of the body. For women with endometriosis, manipulation of the relevant areas can correct any structural problems, encourage pelvic drainage, and reduce uterine congestion.

## Hypnotherapy

Hypnotherapy uses the power of positive suggestion to change your thoughts, feelings or behaviour. A hypnotherapy session will relax your conscious mind while stimulating your subconscious, putting you into a state of heightened awareness while your therapist makes appropriate suggestions, depending on the condition which is being treated. You remain in control the whole time. Relaxation is, of course, very important in the management of pain. When your body is stressed, it tenses up and pain becomes worse. In a hypnotized state you can be taught effective pain management methods which may help with cramps, emotional well-being and fatigue. Anne Lee is a hypnotherapist, psychotherapist and neuro-linguistic programming practitioner who works at the Hale Clinic in London. She says:

> Hypnosis is often not understood. It's an altered state of aware-ness that we all go into many times a day, and hypnotherapists have ways of inducing that state in patients. To help a woman with endometriosis, I would take a really detailed case study of everything that was going on in her life. So much illness starts in the mind and you need to look at every woman as a whole. I would ask how she visualized the endometriosis and how she could practise taking it away. The power of the mind and the imagination is very strong and all I do is give women the respon-sibility for helping their own bodies to heal.

Although the NHS Choices website says there is no strong evi-dence that hypnotherapy works, and studies on the benefits of hypnotherapy tend to be limited and inconclusive, some women do find it helpful. NICE, the National Institute for Health and Care Excellence, has already said hypnotherapy is useful to treat IBS when other treatments have failed – and, of course, it can be used alongside more conventional treatments. If you want to find a reputable hypnotherapist it's a good idea to choose someone who has a background in healthcare and/or is registered with the UK Council for Psychotherapy or the British Society of Clinical and Academic Hypnosis (see Useful addresses). Society members are exclusively health professionals who have done further training in hypnotherapy and use it in their practice.

## Massage

Massage is one of the world's most ancient therapies, dating back to at least 3000 BC and described in texts from China, India, Greece and Rome. It is known to be both physically and mentally soothing. Different techniques are used to manipulate your body's soft tissues with the aim of relieving pain and tension and promoting relaxation. Techniques include effleurage – long, gliding strokes; petrissage – lifting and kneading; and tapotement – tapping.

Almost every country and culture has its own form of massage and it can be confusing to try and find the right one for you. The Hale Clinic in London (see Useful addresses) offers a wide range of complementary therapies and its website <www.haleclinic.com> has information about different forms of massage.

If you have never experienced a massage you might start with the well-known Swedish type, whose aim is to increase the oxygen flow in the blood. It involves moderate pressure and long strokes along the length of the muscles. Swedish massage is recommended for pain and stress reduction and problems with the immune system. Acupressure massage is massage based on the traditional Chinese acupuncture points, but using the hands rather than needles. It can be used to relieve cramps. Shiatsu massage can also help pain control. *Shiatsu* is Japanese for 'finger pressure' and practitioners use touch, comfortable pressure and manipulation to balance the body's energy flow. *Tui Na* is a 2000-year-old Chinese massage technique which uses rhythmic compression to help with associated back pain, stiff neck, and tension headaches.

# 10

# Research

It seems extraordinary that, although endometriosis affects about the same number of women in this country as does diabetes, comparatively little research into endometriosis was being done until the turn of the century. However, Endometriosis UK now reports that this is changing, and since 2000, over 9,700 medical articles have been published on the subject – more than in the previous 45 years! Andrew Horne, Professor of Gynaecology and Reproductive Sciences at Edinburgh University, says that support groups such as Endometriosis UK have to take some of the credit for the heightened awareness of the problem, leading to increases in the amount of research taking place. He says:

> As a condition, it is now being properly recognized by the bodies who fund research. It is being recognized as a burden to society and not just a 'women's health problem' which could be easily dismissed. There are as many women with endometriosis as there are with asthma or diabetes and the social and economic cost in loss of productivity has a major impact. Endometriosis is not just a problem for women, it's a problem for the whole of society. Health conditions which cause pain are invisible, and that has been a problem in the past. It's important for us to educate GPs, and some hospital doctors too, about the condition. Now, though, researchers all over the world are getting together. Last year the EPHect [Endometriosis Phenome and Biobanking Harmonisation Project] guidelines for researchers were published, ensuring that researchers use standardized procedures to collect, process and store tissue samples. Sixteen countries are now involved which means that research can be replicated, resources can be shared, and large-scale research studies will be possible, which is good news.

## Genome-wide association studies

Genome-wide association studies (GWAS) have already proved helpful in identifying the genes associated with inherited forms of breast cancer as well as Crohn's disease and Type 2 diabetes. This technique is a relatively new way to identify the genes involved in particular diseases. Researchers look for tiny variations called SNPs (single nucleotide polymorphisms) which are more common in those with a disease than they are in those without it. This information can then be used to pinpoint genes that may contribute to the risk of developing the disease, and also help to develop strategies to detect, prevent and treat it. Some SNPs have now been identified for endometriosis too, which is a promising development. Associate Professor Krina Zondervan, of the Nuffield Department of Medicine at Oxford University, leads a team of researchers looking at the genetics of endometriosis, including GWAS. She says:

> Our DNA does not change so it can be helpful if variants can be identified. We have been looking at the whole genome rather than the 20,000 individual genes, and comparing women who have endometriosis with those who don't have the condition. We have already identified seven or nine variants and were hoping these would be located on a particular gene, but as yet we have not managed to find out exactly what their function is and what these variants are actually telling us. We have been working with our clinician partners to study actual endometrial tissue from women undergoing laparoscopy operations. Then we shall collect the details from surgical findings and from symptoms and try to integrate the genetic information into the other information we have, to obtain a complete picture. We hope that in a couple of years we will have found more of these genetic signals and that within five years or so, we will understand more about what the signals are telling us.

The doctors and complementary therapists I spoke to agreed that, as far as is known, endometriosis is a multifactorial problem, in that there are lots of different contributory factors which haven't, as yet, been 'joined up' to form a definite cause for endometriosis. As well as assorted causes, the symptoms are very varied, with some women not having any symptoms at all, which is another reason why diagnosis tends to take a long time. As one US researcher put it:

We know that there is a genetic component, an environmental component, and an inflammatory component – but what particular sequence of events leads to particular symptoms? We don't yet know.

It is an encouraging sign that academic researchers, pharmaceutical companies, and doctors themselves are now much more likely to work together and share information.

## Research studies into treatments

An interesting research project at Liverpool Women's Hospital is looking at a particular class of drugs called telomerase inhibitors, which are already being used to treat cancer. Telomerase is an enzyme that 'mends' telomeres, the 'caps' on the end of chromosomes, and research suggests that these drugs may have a potential therapeutic effect on other hormone-related conditions, such as endometriosis. Nicola Tempest, trainee clinical fellow at the Liverpool Women's Hospital, where several different aspects of endometriosis are being studied, says:

> We are looking at women who are having laparoscopic sterilization operations to see whether endometriosis is present so that we have a better idea of how commonly it occurs.
>
> We are also part of a nationwide research project called the Solstice Study which is evaluating a new drug called Elagolix. This is a GnRH antagonist but unlike other drugs of this type it is taken in tablet form and not by injection. At the moment, women are advised not to stay on this type of treatment on a long-term basis because of the risk of developing osteoporosis. We want to find out whether this new drug will be suitable for longer-term use. Currently the trials are at the Phase II stage which means that patients are involved in a research setting. The criteria are quite strict as women in the study must not be taking any kind of hormone treatment such as the pill or a Mirena coil, and they have to be regularly monitored. Techniques for laparoscopic surgery are getting better all the time. In some ways we are having to go back to basics and looking at things like the stem cells in the endometrium to discover whether it is a stem cell problem. Knowing more about the causes of the condition will help researchers to find more effective treatments.

# The need for research

Christian Becker is a gynaecologist and a specialist in reproductive medicine. As well as being Clinical Lead at the Endometriosis Centre in Headington, Oxford, he is an Assistant Professor at Oxford University. His research has focused on biomarkers, which are different characteristics that are used to identify a particular disease or condition. He says:

> At the moment, in order for women to be diagnosed, a laparoscopy has to be performed. It would be much easier if we could diagnose by means of a blood, or saliva, or urine test. Researchers have looked at genetics, various proteins, and cytokines – the latter are chemical messengers secreted by immune cells, which act on other cells to co-ordinate immune responses. Most of the available studies have taken perhaps 30 to 50 women, with the same number in a control group, but there have been no real large-scale studies and the small studies which have been done have sometimes come up with quite different results. There is definitely a need for more large-scale research. Also, we have found that the studies were not standardized and the way samples were collected and processed was not the same, which meant that results varied. Sometimes even the way endometriosis was defined was different in different research studies. However, with the EPHect guidelines, the World Endometriosis Research Foundation has tried to harmonize the way information is collected and processed, including a collaboration between Oxford in the UK and the University of Harvard in the USA. At least we now have a standard and we know everyone is doing the same thing, and there is certainly no shortage of patients out there!
>
> One recent finding has made us think that the various different entities within endometriosis might actually have different origins. That means that lesions in the peritoneal cavity might have a different origin from chocolate cysts or nodules which develop on the bowel or bladder. There doesn't seem to be much correlation between the amount of endometriosis present, and the severity of a woman's symptoms. We know that retrograde menstruation is involved but it is normal for women to experience this. One theory is that in some women the cells are over-expressing certain enzymes which then adhere to other organs. Sometimes, we can see this happening. But there are no definite answers yet.

Fertility is an issue too, of course. About a third to a half of women with endometriosis have fertility problems – but endometriosis doesn't necessarily interfere with fertility. Perhaps, in some women, the endometrial tissue is different in some way that makes it more difficult for a fertilized embryo to implant? We just don't yet know.

The role of the immune system is being researched in this country, in the USA and in Belgium. Macrophages, which are a type of white blood cell which can swallow up invading bacteria and play a critical role in immune regulation, can be dysfunctional and may not be expressing cytokines – or, on the other hand, they may be producing something which encourages blood vessels to grow. Lesions do not always cause pain, so is it the inflammation which actually does cause the pain? Again, we don't yet know.

If the actual causes of endometriosis are not yet clear, what is the picture as regards new treatments? Dr Becker says that most existing treatments are hormone based, in one way or another, which means there is a risk of side effects, some more serious than others. He says:

> All drugs tend to work in a similar way whether they are taken in the form of a pill, a patch or injections. As clinicians we have to work with what is available. Given the choices we have at the moment, I would always choose the drug with the fewest side effects for every individual. Of course I discuss the treatment options with patients. For example, if the pill has not helped her I might offer her a Mirena coil. It is very much a matter of trial and error and women need to be patient and aware of the issues involved. They may never be totally pain-free, but there is help out there.

Dr Becker also points out that it is important, not just for the individuals concerned, but for society as a whole, that solutions are found.

> Endometriosis, especially if it is severe, affects a woman's whole life including her relationships and her sex life. There is a cost perspective too. It's not just the price of drugs and surgery and hospital stays, it's the cost to society of employing women who can't work effectively because they are so ill. Pharmaceutical

companies are trying to provide non-hormone-based treatments because the side effects of some of the existing ones can be a problem. They are also working on treatments for pregnant women who are not able to take current medications. The new Bayer pill, Visanne, especially formulated to treat endometriosis, seems to be quite successful in the European countries where it has been used but it is expensive. There have also been a couple of trials of new injectable drugs, but as far as I am aware no ground-breaking treatment is likely to emerge in the next couple of years. Bearing in mind most new drugs are in development for 10 to 15 years, I think we are stuck with what we have for the moment. A drug specifically for endometriosis, which has few side effects for the majority, would change so many women's lives.

## Non-hormonal treatment

Professor Horne, of Edinburgh University, agrees that a non-hormonal treatment, which could be taken safely by young women who wanted to become pregnant and which did not cause side effects, would be the gold standard of treatments. Of the existing treatments, all surgery carries risks, which is why finding an effective non-surgical treatment would be beneficial. It's also true that some 20–50 per cent of women in the UK, and some 20–40 per cent in the US, who have surgery to treat endometriosis, tend to get a recurrence of the problem within five years. The medical treatments, such as the mini-pill or Depo-Provera or the GnRH analogues, all have side effects, and when women stop taking them the symptoms recur. Professor Horne's area of interest is non-hormonal treatments, and something he has been looking at is the role of omega-3 fatty acids. These are known to have an impact on pain and anti-inflammatory properties, and they reduce lesions in animals. Some trials have been done in Edinburgh, and when Professor Horne and his team asked for volunteers through Endometriosis UK, 600 women came forward. Many of them were taking omega-3 supplements already and were finding them helpful. Professor Horne is hoping a suitable dietary supplement will be found, or perhaps existing drugs, which are used to reduce pain in other conditions, will be found to help treat endometriosis.

# 11

# Support and help

The effect of endometriosis on quality of life shouldn't be under-estimated. A recent major international study by the World Endometriosis Research Foundation looked at almost one thousand women in ten different countries and found that:

- 51 per cent reported that their work was affected by endometriosis;
- 50 per cent reported that their relationships were affected;
- over 50 per cent reported painful sex;
- 60 per cent reported chronic pelvic pain;
- women reported reduced quality of life in all areas, including childcare, exercise, housework, shopping and study.

In addition, there is the cost of such a high rate of chronic sickness to the National Health Service and the economy. Recently this was estimated at a whopping £8.2 billion in treatment, loss of work days and healthcare costs. So, if you suspect that endometriosis might be at the root of your problems and you haven't yet obtained a diagnosis, or you have been diagnosed but are not sure where to go from here, what can you do?

## Endometriosis UK

One source of help is Endometriosis UK (see Useful addresses). This is a small charity whose aim is to help women take back control of their health. The helpline number is 0808 808 2227. The helpline is staffed by volunteers so opening times vary but you can check this out on the website. Endometriosis UK provides free and reli-able information about symptoms, treatments, and current research into endometriosis and above all, support from women who know exactly what the problems can be. Whether you are especially con-cerned about pain, the impact endometriosis has on your working life or family life or sex life, or whether you want up-to-date advice on fertility issues, they are the people who can offer support. If you are looking for local support, or simply someone to talk to, you may find there are groups near you who run regular meetings, as well as fundraising events and social get-togethers. If there's nothing within reach you might consider starting one up, as many of the volunteers who run local groups have done!

## Other online support

Online support is also available via a forum available at <https://healthunlocked.com/endometriosis-uk>. Go online and you will find women telling their own stories and asking for advice on every possible endometriosis-related issue. Some are newly diagnosed, others have been coping with endometriosis for years. If you want to know how to convince your partner that you're not rejecting him just because you can't face having agonizingly painful sex, or you are ready to give up hope of having a baby, there will be other women on the forum who can reassure you and wish you luck – and, yes, there *are* happy endings to some of the stories posted!

One of Endometriosis UK's other main aims is to raise awareness of endometriosis among health professionals – the evidence shows that some women are still being told that severe period pain is 'just part of being a woman' – and also among the general public, including, of course, the families, partners and friends of women who have endometriosis. They also support research into the causes of, and treatments for, endometriosis. Many of the women interviewed for this book said they had never heard of endometriosis and that, if they had, they would have mentioned it to their GP when they first consulted him or her about severe period pain or other symptoms.

ITV's *This Morning* programme held an Endometriosis Awareness Week in March 2014 with the support of Endometriosis UK. Their spokeswomen pointed out that endometriosis can wreck lives and relationships and is a leading cause of infertility, so the condition really should be better known. A year later there was a Worldwide Endo March in London in another attempt to raise awareness. There has also been celebrity support. Singer Dolly Parton, actress Anna Friel and former Spice Girl Emma Bunton have all suffered from endometriosis in the past. TV presenters Carol Smillie and

Annabel Croft have even started the 'Diary Doll' company producing specially designed pants with a 'discreet' waterproof panel,
suitable for girls and women who need extra reassurance that they
won't be embarrassed by leakage or flooding. More information can
be obtained from their website <www.diarydoll.com>.

Experts and women with endometriosis all say the same
thing – 'Keep pestering the health professionals until they listen!'
If you aren't happy with what your GP can tell you – and remember
that GPs can't be experts in every condition they're presented with
– then ask for a second opinion or a referral to one of the specialist
Endometriosis Centres.

## Endometriosis Centres

The British Society for Gynaecological Endoscopy (see Useful
addresses), which is part of the Royal College of Obstetricians
and Gynaecologists, has been instrumental in setting up accredited Endometriosis Centres all over the UK. There are now about
30 of these and if you are referred to one you may be able to
see any member of a multi-disciplinary team of gynaecologists,
specialist nurses, colo-rectal surgeons, urologists and pain management specialists, depending on your individual needs. Christian
Becker is Clinical Lead at the Endometriosis Centre in Headington,
Oxford. This is the second largest centre in the country and, as
required by the government, is accredited by the British Society for
Gynaecological Endoscopy (BSGE). The idea of setting up these specialist centres is that women with severe endometriosis could then
be treated by clinicians with appropriate expertise. Dr Becker says:

> Women are referred to us from all over the country by their GPs.
> Usually they come to us because the treatment they have received
> from their GP has not helped and they may also have fertility
> problems linked to the condition. I generally ask them which
> is more important for them at this moment in time – is it the
> pain, or are they trying to get pregnant and having problems?
> Then we proceed with treatment for whichever is more impor-
> tant to the patient. Clinics are held weekly and we have weekly
> meetings with colleagues to discuss treatment options. I'll be
> speaking to nurses, pain specialists, perhaps colo-rectal surgeons

and urologists. We might decide on further investigations such as an MRI scan, or, if the woman has already had investigations, we might offer hormonal pain treatment or possibly surgery. I've been involved in creating European-wide guidelines on treatments. If a particular patient's main worries are about fertility – as well as the pain she is suffering – I might suggest a laparoscopy and either burning – with a laser – or cutting out the lesions. If the woman says she doesn't want surgery then I might suggest a course of IVF, if she has been trying to become pregnant without success for a year or two.

The benefits of attending a centre like ours are the multi-disciplinary approach. We have expert nurses who are the first point of contact. We have gynaecologists who can operate – we do about 60 operations a year – colo-rectal surgeons who step in if there are adhesions to the bowel, and urologists whose expertise is concerned with the bladder and kidneys. Not forgetting the pain specialists who can offer help in managing the pain on a day-to-day basis. We probably see about ten new patients in the clinic every week. Some are referred to us from other clinics. In very severe cases where there are complex conditions involving the bladder and bowel or other organs, we will ask women to fill in a detailed questionnaire about exactly how the condition affects every aspect of their life. We offer follow up appointments after six months and welcome feedback at any time. One of our specialist nurses will call patients around six to eight weeks after surgery to see how they are getting on, and women know they can come back to us if they have problems. It's very important with this chronic condition that we are an approachable team.

Most of the women we see are between their mid-20s and the menopause, but I have run clinics for teenagers too. We have also organized a day to raise awareness of the condition among GPs. One GP actually asked us if we weren't running the risk of labelling all period pains endometriosis and suggested that women should just deal with it! This is probably why it takes women so long to be diagnosed and treated. It's not a condition women die from and on the whole it's not one that is much talked about – but it still affects a lot of women's lives!

## Rosemary

Rosemary, whose condition was much improved by regular acupuncture sessions as we saw in Chapter 8, says that it was almost by chance that she was diagnosed at all!

> I had tried several GPs as I'd moved house a lot, but they were really dismissive and I got the impression I would just have to put up with my heavy and painful periods. Perhaps I was just unlucky? Eventually, I had some pre-cancerous cells removed after a smear test and happened to see a lovely consultant who felt my tummy and said 'You have endometriosis'! It was all over my lower abdomen and seemed to be attached to most of my organs.

> I had several operations, hormone injections and tried a Mirena coil, but nothing seemed to help. I was also told I would not be able to get pregnant. I had one ectopic pregnancy and then, to my great surprise, became pregnant again in 2001. Ironically, I felt amazing while I was expecting – the best I have ever felt. I really blossomed and felt healthy for about the first time ever. I had the acupuncture, which helped a lot, but also tried to help myself. I most definitely think that diet makes a difference. Sugar, caffeine and alcohol can make the symptoms worse. I did go and see a dietician to see what she would recommend. Although going organic can be expensive, it does help. I like to use farm shops and buy locally grown produce. I found out what suited me by trial and error. I don't eat too much fruit because it contains sugar, but I do eat a lot of green vegetables.

> It's hard to feel good about yourself when you feel battered and bruised. When I had migraines I became terribly tired which is no fun if, like me, you are an active person. I found that if I was fuelled by the right food, I could get out and about. I took up running, which helps with moods because it balances your hormones. I also do yoga which I use for relaxation and to centre me if I am feeling grumpy and fed up. I no longer let endometriosis rule my life!

## Other sources of help

It's worth remembering that you can get help for chronic pain on the NHS, whatever the condition that causes it. Chronic pain – which is usually defined as pain which lasts for three months or more – is a complex subject and can, as we know, be hard to treat effectively. Some women are simply offered stronger and stronger painkillers, which may or may not work and may also have side effects if taken in the long term. A better solution may be pain management, which teaches you how to live your life in spite of the pain – to control it rather than letting it control you. Ask yourself what your pain is getting in the way of, what you'd like to do to help yourself and how your partner, family, friends and colleagues could help you cope.

Long-term, chronic pain often arises from conditions such as endometriosis which are not yet fully understood. As the experts quoted earlier in the book have said, we don't yet know why some women suffer from severe pain while others don't. In the meantime it might be possible for you to be referred to a pain clinic. There are about 300 of these all over the country, usually attached to hospitals, and staffed by a multi-disciplinary team of experts including doctors and psychologists. To access a pain clinic you will need to be referred by your GP. You might also benefit by contacting the British Pain Society (see Useful addresses) who can tell you where your nearest pain clinic can be found.

As well as discussing painkilling drugs and injections, pain clinics may offer alternatives including, interestingly, such complementary treatments as acupuncture and hypnotherapy (see Chapter 9 for more information on these). Pain management sessions are a kind of group therapy, usually for 6–8 people, teaching special physical, psychological and practical techniques to help improve your quality of life. The British Pain Society also offers a booklet called *Understanding and Managing Pain*, which is downloadable from their website.

## Help and support for relationship problems

With about half of women with endometriosis reporting that sex is painful for them, it's clear that endometriosis has a huge impact on many relationships. World Endometriosis Research Foundation (see Useful addresses) studies show that, like many aspects of endometriosis, the pain women suffer and the problems it causes vary. Some women report sharp, stabbing pains during intercourse, others mention a deep ache which can continue for as long as 24 or 48 hours afterwards, or even both. Sometimes deep penetration is unbearable, some women can't tolerate sex during a period, others find it painful at any time of the month. The technical name for painful sex is dyspareunia and the severity of the pain may depend on where in your body the endometriosis lesions and nodules are found – possibly behind your vagina or around the lower end of your uterus. Some of the hormone treatments for endometriosis can result in a medically induced menopause and a dry and sensitive vagina, as can the after-effects of a hysterectomy.

The WERF experts recommend open and honest communication between partners when painful sex is a problem. Both you and your partner might feel fear, guilt, resentment or a mixture of these and it's vital to talk about it so that you both know you're dealing with a painful physical condition and it's not about lack of love or a relationship which is going wrong! Relate counsellor and sex therapist Denise Knowles says:

> Endometriosis is like an unwelcome lodger in some couples' and families' lives. Women don't mean to make life a misery for their partners and families – not to mention themselves – but if they are in chronic pain, possibly sleep-deprived, it can impact their whole lives. I remember counselling a woman who was a nurse and worked shifts, who had to tell her employers there were two or three days every month when she just couldn't work. A chronic condition like this impacts on so many areas as well as affecting how women feel about themselves as women and as sexual beings.
>
> Having a diagnosis can help because then women and their partners at least know what they are dealing with, and can begin to negotiate around it. Being able to talk about it is vital. I am always amazed how many couples find it hard to talk about their sexual relationships. Many, too, think that penetration is the only kind of real sex. There are other ways to be sensual, intimate and loving.
>
> Couples also have to learn to manage disappointment if they can't have sex the way they want to. For instance if a woman is bleeding heavily she may not feel 'clean' enough for oral sex. Sometimes women with endometriosis find the contractions of orgasm painful too. But if they withdraw from any sort of

contact the partner feels rejected and abandoned, perhaps even suspicious. I would always say – talk about it, and what it means to you. Admit you are disappointed and then work out ways of being close and loving which are still possible. The unknown is always scary and our imaginations always take us to the darkest place, rather than seeing endometriosis as a problem you both have and can work on. Therapy can help by working towards a mutual understanding.

There's a message for other family members and friends too. Because endometriosis is not much talked about, even other women tend to dismiss it as 'just period pain' without understanding. If friends realize that this is a chronic condition which is inconvenient and frustrating and involves arranging a woman's working and social life around her periods – because of a pain that may be a hundred times worse than a straightforward period cramp – then they may be more supportive!

Consultant gynaecologist Caroline Overton adds:

Try and get on with your life as well as you can. Take painkillers if you need to, sticking to paracetamol with or without ibuprofen, and keeping the stronger painkillers for a flare-up. You can develop a tolerance to the stronger painkillers when they can appear to stop working, so once the pain from the flare-up starts to ease, try cutting out the stronger drugs again. Make sure you eat a balanced diet with plenty of fresh fruit and vegetables. If you do try a special diet, make sure it contains all the essential nutrients and vitamins you need. If you can get past the tiredness, exercise can really help because it releases the endorphins which are the body's natural painkillers.

# Useful addresses

## General

**Endometriosis SHE Trust UK**
Website: http://shetrust.org.uk

**Endometriosis UK**
Helpline: 0808 808 2227
Website: www.endometriosis-uk.org
Support and campaign group for women affected by the condition.

**World Endometriosis Research Foundation**
Website: http://endometriosisfoundation.org

## Support for managing symptoms and related conditions

**Adenomyosis Advice Association**
Website: www.adenomyosisadviceassociation.org
Support for women with the related condition adenomyosis.

**British Pain Society**
Website: www.britishpainsociety.org
Advice, information and support for those managing pain.

**British Society for Gynaecological Endoscopy**
Website: http://bsge.org.uk
Promotes the benefits of minimal access or keyhole surgery as a way of treating women with gynaecological problems including endometriosis. It also has a list of nationwide-registered endometriosis centres where women can receive specialist treatment.

**Core**
Tel.: 020 7486 0341
Website: www.corecharity.org.uk
Support and information for people with digestive disorders.

**Crohn's and Colitis UK**
Helpline: 0845 130 2233
Website: www.crohnsandcolitis.org.uk
Information and support for people with inflammatory bowel disorders.

**Hysterectomy Association**
Website: www.hysterectomy-association.org.uk

**IBS Network**
Tel.: 0114 272 3253
Website: www.theibsnetwork.org
Information and support for people with irritable bowel syndrome. Offers a helpline to members.

**Maryon Stewart**
Tel. (appointments): 07921 417432
Website: www.maryonstewart.com
For advice on nutritional approaches to managing endometriosis (and other gynaecological conditions).

**Pelvic Pain Support Network**
Website: http://pelvicpain.org.uk
Information about conditions that cause pelvic pain.

**Relate**
Helpline: 0300 100 1234
Website: www.relate.org.uk
Offers help with all kinds of relationship problems.

**UK Council for Psychotherapy**
Website: www.ukcp.org.uk

## Fertility and adoption

**Adoption UK**
Helpline: 0844 848 7900 (10 a.m. to 4 p.m., Monday to Friday)
Website: www.adoptionuk.org
A support group for adopters and those planning to adopt, run by and for adopters.

**First4Adoption**
Website: www.first4adoption.org.uk
Information about adoption and about children looking for new families.

**Fertility Fairness**
Website: www.fertilityfairness.co.uk
A group that campaigns for better access to fertility treatment.

**Human Fertilisation and Embryology Authority (HFEA)**
Website: www.hfea.gov.uk
Information about fertility treatment and clinics.

**Infertility Network UK**
Helpline: 0800 008 7464
Website: www.infertilitynetworkuk.com
Up-to-date information on infertility.

## Complementary therapies

**Acumedic Centre**
Website: www.acumedic.com
Long-established North London centre for Chinese medicine.

**Association of Reflexologists**
Website: www.aor.org.uk
Information about reflexology and details of local therapists.

**British Acupuncture Council**
Website: www.acupuncture.org.uk
Information about acupuncture and help to a find local practitioner.

**British Autogenic Society**
Website: www.autogenic-therapy.org.uk
Information about autogenic therapy and local therapists.

**British Homeopathic Association**
Tel.: 01582 408675
Website: www.britishhomeopathic.org
Information about homoeopathy and details of local practitioners.

**British Society of Clinical and Academic Hypnosis**
Website: www.bscah.com
Information and advice on finding a hypnotherapist.

**British Wheel of Yoga**
Website: www.bwy.org.uk
Details of yoga teachers and classes around the UK.

**General Osteopathic Council**
Website: www.osteopathy.org.uk
Information and details of local osteopaths.

**Hale Clinic**
Tel.: 020 7631 0156
Website: www.haleclinic.com
An established complementary medical clinic offering a variety of
treatments, including hypnotherapy and massage.

**Judy Elliott, acupuncturist and fertility coach**
Tel.: 07885 226603
Website: www.judith-elliott.com

**Mindfulness and online mindfulness courses**
Website: http://bemindful.co.uk

**National Institute of Medical Herbalists**
Website: www.nimh.org.uk
Information about medical herbalists all over the UK.

**Tracey Smith, reflexologist**
Tel.: 01823 364952

# References

1 Sinaii N, Cleary SD, Ballweg ML et al. High rates of autoimmune and endocrine disorders, fibromyalgia, chronic fatigue syndrome and atopic diseases among women with endometriosis: a survey analysis. *Human Reproduction* 2002; 17(10): 2715–24.

2 Nnoaham KE, Hummelshoj L, Webster P et al. Impact of endometriosis on quality of life and work productivity: a multicenter study across ten countries. *Fertility and Sterility* 2011; 96(2): 366–73.

3 Andersen MR, Goff BA, Lowe KA. Development of an instrument to identify symptoms potentially indicative of ovarian cancer in a primary care clinic setting. *Open Journal of Obstetrics and Gynecology* 2012; 2(3): 183–191.

4 Grodstein F, Goldman MB, Ryan L, Cramer DW. Relation of female infertility to consumption of caffeinated beverages. *American Journal of Epidemiology* 1993; 137(12): 1353–60.

5 Parazzini F, Chiaffarini F, Surace M et al. Selected food intake and risk of endometriosis. *Human Reproduction* 2004; 19(8): 1755–9.

6 Dhillon PK, Holt VL. Recreational physical activity and endometrioma risk. *American Journal of Epidemiology* 2003; 13(6): 392–3.

7 Barbieri RL. Etiology and epidemiology of endometriosis. *American Journal of Obstetrics and Gynecology* 1990; 16(2): 565–7.

8 Kold M et al. Mindfulness-based psychological intervention for coping with pain in endometriosis. *Nordic Psychology* 2012; 64(1): 2–16.

9 Reiner K, Tibi L, Lipsitz JD. Mindful practices – do mindfulness-based interventions reduce pain intensity? A critical review of the literature. *Pain Medicine* 2013; 14(2): 230–42.

# Index

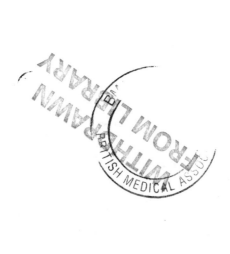
WITHDRAWN FROM LIBRARY

BRITISH MEDICAL ASSOC